HAWTHORNS CHILDRENS

Penguin Books
My Child Won't

Elisabeth Morse is a qualified nutritionist and was a member of the working group that produced the well-known NACNE report. She is also a well-established journalist who has written articles for women's magazines, medical newspapers and several of the Open University health education courses.

Elisabeth Morse

MY CHILD WON'T EAT

Penguin Books

To my sons Christopher and Matthew, who have
taught me more about putting the theory of nutrition
into practice than any textbook can ever do

PENGUIN BOOKS

Published by the Penguin Group
27 Wrights Lane, London W 8 5 T Z, England
Viking Penguin Inc., 40 West 23rd Street, New York, New York 10010, U S A
Penguin Books Australia Ltd, Ringwood, Victoria, Australia
Penguin Books Canada Ltd, 2801 John Street, Markham, Ontario, Canada L 3 R 1 B 4
Penguin Books (N Z) Ltd, 182–190 Wairau Road, Auckland 10, New Zealand

Penguin Books Ltd, Registered Offices: Harmondsworth, Middlesex, England

First published 1988

Copyright © Elisabeth Morse, 1988
All rights reserved

Made and printed in Great Britain by
Richard Clay Ltd, Bungay, Suffolk
Filmset in Linotron Trump by
Rowland Phototypesetting Ltd, Bury St Edmunds, Suffolk

Contents

Chapter 1
Introduction

The chances are you have bought this book because you have a child who either eats little or won't eat the foods you think he or she ought to eat. It is important to realize that you are not alone: about a quarter of all children under five are described by their parents as poor eaters. Some parents are able to shrug off their children's apparent eating problems as 'just a phase', but not everyone feels so confident. The desire to feed one's child is a very powerful instinct, so it is not surprising if the parents of a child who 'won't eat' feel vulnerable. It is quite understandable that they equate not eating with being ill or interpret it as a form of hunger strike – thoughts that can trigger strong emotional reactions of anxiety and anger – but a child with a poor appetite is, in fact, behaving like many other well-adjusted, healthy children.

Food fads and quirks of appetite are very much a part of normal growth and development. Understanding what is normal behaviour and how your child acquires practical skills can help you put many of the so-called problems into perspective. Eating problems sometimes arise because parents expect too much or too little of a child. Readjusting your expectations so that they are realistic, and understanding the sorts of problems that are common, will help you not only to cope when problems do occur, but also to prevent them from arising.

Occasionally an appetite problem that looks like a normal food fad is caused by ill health, but there is usually little difficulty in telling the difference between a healthy (though possibly cross) child and a sickly one who needs medical attention. The majority of children with food problems are healthy, and, with normal care and attention, should grow out of a period of eating difficulties. Sometimes, however, a phase can become a habit; but even bad habits can be broken with a little planning and good management.

A feeding problem can arise suddenly, but most develop gradually over several weeks or months. Sometimes feeding problems are present from birth, and although they are different in many ways from those that arise at the toddler stage, if your confidence has been shaken right from the beginning, feeding your child may continue to be especially difficult for you.

Most eating problems are caused by a clash of wills – even if you don't want a battle, your child will probably be trying to provoke one. You know from your own and others' experience that such clashes are an inevitable part of the growing-up process. They play an important role in helping a child find out where the limits to his behaviour are set. Finding out where the line is drawn helps a child feel secure and cared for, but knowing where to set those limits is not always an easy task for parents.

This book explains the stages your child is likely to go through in developing eating habits and gives you practical advice on how to tackle the problems that can arise. It assumes that the parent most involved and concerned with feeding a child is the mother, whether she is at home or goes out to work. However, this book is intended for whichever parent has the responsibility for seeing that the child is fed. (In my experience fathers, like nannies and child-minders, tend to take a more sanguine approach to a child's poor eating habits and feel – probably correctly – that worry is likely only to make the problem worse!)

Although the first seven chapters concern specific age groups, many eating problems can occur at different ages. Details about the method of management may vary somewhat depending on the age of the child, but the fundamental principles remain the same. The problems dealt with are the common ones, such as weaning difficulties, food fads, poor appetite and, later, differences of opinon about which foods are acceptable. The management of such problems, although worrying to parents, does not usually elicit the same degree of concern from family doctors, who frequently tell anxious parents simply 'not to worry, let the child eat what he or she wants, and the problem will go away eventually'. This often is true, but it can be very difficult to follow such advice unless you know *why* you need not worry, *what* sorts of foods can be offered freely without risk to health and *how long* a problem is likely to continue before it resolves itself – all questions that this book sets out to answer.

In addition, there are chapters on healthy eating for children, the overweight child and food allergies. Eating problems may arise not only when a child refuses foods, but also when a parent refuses to give a child certain foods in the belief that they may be 'bad' for him. And although this book is about children who do not eat, overweight children are included because they can suffer from similar eating problems. A great deal of publicity is given to food allergies, the causes of overweight and what constitutes a healthy diet for a child, and it is important to sort out the facts from the mis-information and prejudice when deciding how to cope with your child's day-to-day eating problems.

It is also important to know what this book does *not*

include. It does not discuss the dietary management of organic and metabolic disorders, as children with such problems will be under specialist medical care and supervision. Nor does it discuss children with severe growth disorders, because their small stature is more usually the result of hormonal insufficiency than a shortage of food. Anorexia nervosa is not discussed in detail because it is a rare disorder of adolescence and even rarer in younger children.

The advice in this book is aimed at resolving your child's eating problems in ways that allow him freedom and independence within clearly defined limits so that he – and you – know that *you* are in charge – even if that does not always mean the same as complete control! The suggestions have been gleaned mainly from those who have had to deal with food problems: doctors, health visitors and, mostly, other parents.

Chapter 2
The new-born baby

One of the most surprising discoveries for parents when their first child is born is that this tiny, helpless bundle is as capable of affecting the household as a fully grown adult coming to stay. A baby's needs seem simple enough in theory, but making sure his tummy is comfortably full, that he gets all the sleep he wants and feels snuggly and warm is not always easy in practice. You will spend a lot of time feeding your baby in the early weeks of his life. Feeds can often take an hour or more, and some babies need feeding every two to three hours or even more frequently, which leaves you little time to do much else.

A healthy baby has no difficulty in letting you know when he is not comfortable: he will cry, very often with an intensity that any parent may have great difficulty in ignoring for more than a couple of minutes! Since feeding is a new-born baby's main activity, it is not surprising if you interpret his cries as a sign of hunger. Checking that he is getting enough milk is a sensible start; if he is, hunger is unlikely to be the cause. Babies can cry for all sorts of reasons and, it should be realized, for no apparent reason at all. Many mothers will testify that they had thriving babies who were kept clean, cuddled and rested, but who nevertheless had spells of crying, which eventually stopped for as little reason as they began.

Is your baby healthy?

Healthy, thriving babies have warm, silky skins, and their flesh is firm and elastic. When awake, they are alert, looking around and taking an interest in what is going on and, particularly, in other people. They move and kick well, showing surprising strength for those so little. They sleep soundly, but there is little difficulty waking them when it is time for a feed. Healthy babies wet their nappies regularly throughout the day, though the amount they dirty them can vary enormously from once a week to several times a day. Some babies frequently spit up small amounts of partially digested milk after feeds and are described as 'sicky' babies.

Babies who are underfed or ill tend to sleep for long periods, are persistently difficult to wake for a feed, are sleepy feeders, seem listless and apathetic when awake *and* have poor weight gains. Babies with these symptoms need medical attention. Even a minor infection can make a baby sleepy, and a slight cold or soreness can make it difficult for a baby to feed or sleep properly.

All healthy new-born babies *want* to eat, but some find it difficult to feed. These feeding problems are very different from those that are likely to develop in the older baby and young child, and are not an indicator of a mother's ability to care for her child. Although it is highly unlikely that a baby will remember these early difficulties, many parents will and, as a result, may suffer a real blow to their confidence from the very beginning. Such feelings of guilt are perhaps experienced most acutely by the woman who fully intended to breast-feed her baby but had little success.

Difficulties in establishing breast-feeding

Although there is a wide range of feeding problems that can occur in the early weeks of life, they probably all stem from three different – but often related – sources. Firstly, there may be insufficient stimulation of the milk supply; the responsibility for this is as much the midwife's as the mother's. Secondly, there may be physical problems: the mother might have sore nipples, or the baby might suffer from severe crying spells. Thirdly, the parents might have particular difficulty in accepting and adjusting to the fact that having a baby means an enormous change in their lives. For all these reasons breast-feeding may be abandoned in favour of the bottle.

The milk supply

A baby is born with a number of reflex actions. For example, if his cheek is touched, he will instinctively and immediately turn towards the touch and root for the nipple. If a nipple, teat or finger is then put in his mouth, he will automatically start to suck, and if liquid is sucked, he will swallow it. These reflexes are strongest in the first few hours after birth. If the new-born baby is given the opportunity to feed in these first hours and thereafter every three to four hours, his rooting, sucking and swallowing reflexes will remain strong for about the next three months. By the end of this period he will have learnt what food is for and he won't need to be stimulated to feed by the action of his automatic reflexes.

The newly delivered mother begins to produce breast milk, stimulated by hormones released by the act of giving birth and by the action of the baby sucking. The milk is released into milk sacs behind the nipple in response to what is known as the let-down reflex. After a few days, when the breasts are beginning to make larger quantities of milk, some mothers feel this reflex as a tingling sensation in the breast.

If the baby's or the mother's reflexes are not stimulated, they can weaken. A baby who is prevented from sucking and feeding in the first twelve hours or so of life – maybe because he is ill, has been given a bottle or is sleepy from drugs given to the mother during labour – may develop a poor sucking response. Such babies can be slow, difficult feeders. They may find a bottle, which requires less vigorous sucking than a nipple, easier to feed from than the breast.

A mother whose breasts are insufficiently stimulated by a baby with poor sucking action may not only find it difficult to produce enough milk, but may also become increasingly discouraged at the baby's slow response. If she is upset, exhausted or even embarrassed, her let-down reflex may also be inhibited so that little or no milk is produced. For these reasons, complementary feeds (bottles of milk formula that are given as supplements to breast milk) can often bring about the end of breast-feeding.

If these reflexes have been partly inhibited, establishing satisfactory breast-feeding will require determination and support. Some mothers feel that the extra effort required is not worth the possible misery when alternative, highly sophisticated milk formulas are available. But if you are determined to try to breast-feed, the sooner you tackle the problem of an insufficient milk supply, the better. This means spending two or three days (or even more, if necessary) concentrating only on feeding, so that you allow the baby plenty of time at the breast – waking him if necessary – and do little yourself besides eating, sleeping and feeding him.

If the baby tires quickly from sucking and needs to be given milk from a bottle, you could try giving him milk expressed from your breasts with a breast pump, as this will help stimulate your milk supply. In the beginning tiredness and inexperience can make it difficult to work out problems and you may need the support and guidance of someone who is used to coping with such problems. This could be either a midwife or a breast-feeding counsellor (a mother who has successfully breast-fed and who has been trained to help others) from the National Childbirth Trust (see p. 132).

Physical difficulties

Having a plentiful milk supply is a tremendous confidence booster, but, unfortunately, does not necessarily mean the end of all problems. Sore, and even cracked, nipples can be common in the early days and, later, a blocked milk duct can cause discomfort. These problems are perhaps not surprising given the fact that in Britain most women wear close-fitting nylon bras, which encourage nipples to be soft and delicate rather than strong and elastic. Again, the sooner these problems are tackled, the sooner they will go away.

In most cases, a change in feeding position is needed to ensure that the baby has the nipple well inside his mouth. Lying down on your side to feed the baby or sitting up and holding him under one arm rather than across your lap will help take the pressure off the sore parts and give them a chance to recover.

You should wash your nipples just once a day and with water only, as soap tends to remove the natural oils that are present. You need to keep your nipples dry between feeds. Ideally this means letting the air get to them so that any drips of milk can evaporate quickly. A cotton feeding-bra allows air to circulate and so is preferable to a nylon one, which does not. Breast creams and sprays are available, but whether they help or even prolong the problem is uncertain.

If there is nothing wrong with your nipples or your milk supply, but your baby seems to be sick a lot or have severe crying spells, you may find yourself questioning the suitability of your milk. Do not worry: a mother's milk is almost always suitable for her baby. It is quite normal for babies to frequently spit up or regurgitate small quantities of milk and even occasionally to throw up what looks like a whole feed. Provided the baby seems well otherwise and is gaining weight satisfactorily, there is nothing to be alarmed about. Being sick is not usually distressing for a baby – it is just messy for you! To minimize the problem be especially careful to handle your baby gently and, perhaps, shorten the length of the feed so that he does not get too full.

Crying for no apparent reason is a problem that can be very distressing for both you and the baby, and it is not easy to cure. You may try every imaginable solution, but not try any one for long enough in your anxiety to stop the crying as soon as possible. Assuming that the baby is comfortably warm (you can test this by putting your finger down the back of his neck to see if his skin feels the same temperature as yours) and has had a nappy change fairly recently, the first thing to try is giving him some milk. If a little sucking is followed by crying, then it may be that he wants milk and can't get it or that he wants to suck without feeding. If your baby is gaining weight well, the former is unlikely to be the problem. If he wants only the sucking action, try giving him your little finger with the soft side uppermost or a dummy.

If sucking or feeding are not the answer, try holding

your baby upright against your shoulder and gently patting and rocking or walking him about. Imposing a soothing rhythm on his cries should help calm you even if it does not soothe him instantly, and if you feel calmer, you will be better able to help him. Having his tummy supported firmly and in an upright position will also help ease any tummy pain as well as making it easier for him to burp up any air he has swallowed while crying. If the wind is all down at the other end, lay him on his stomach across your knee and rhythmically pat his bottom. If, like some babies, he cries when he is tired, being supported in a gentle rocking movement, perhaps in a position close enough to hear your heart beat, may send him off to sleep.

If the crying spells regularly begin at a particular time of day, such as the late afternoon or evening, and if the baby screams for two to twenty minutes at a time, he may have colic. Remarkably, this sort of crying stops at about as regular a time as it begins and usually disappears at around three months. If the colic is particularly bad, a breast-feeding mother may be advised to eliminate all dairy foods from her diet. If you decide to try this approach, consult your doctor first and then follow the diet for only two weeks; that is long enough to find out whether it is working or not. Cutting out milk, butter, cheese and eggs and all foods containing them is not easy. Not only does it mean a very restricted diet, but there is no guarantee that it will work; only about one-third of babies are helped in this way.

Colicky babies are usually thriving in every other way. If your baby is putting on plenty of weight and growing well, you could try to establish a more definite routine of feeding and sleeping, as there is some evidence that colicky babies respond to this. You will probably feel better, too, if you have more of a pattern in your daily life, with regular spells of fresh air, play times with your baby and times when you can have a bit of peace and quiet on your own. A strict routine can be restricting and does not appeal to everyone. It is a good idea to discuss your particular needs and work out a suitable timetable with someone else, such as your health visitor.

A period of adjustment

Some parents need to allow themselves more time to adjust to the presence of a baby. You can't expect to continue to follow your former way of life, particularly if it was busy and demanding, without making some changes. At first you might feel that the relationship is all 'take' on the part of the baby, but after the first month or two, when he starts to smile and laugh, you will discover that he has a great deal to give as well. And once you start to realize the rewards, you may find that it makes a fundamental change to your perspective on life.

Having a baby is like starting a new job and, as in any new job, you may feel unsure from time to time as you gradually find out what is needed of you and learn to cope. Just what is needed of each set of parents is a very individual matter. It depends not only on your particular circumstances, but also on the personality and specific requirements of your baby. You may be happier if you try to be flexible and cater for what both you and your baby actually need than if you try, often in vain, to make life the way you imagine it ought to be. For example, some parents find that their baby won't fit into a regular routine of feeding and sleeping (as grandmothers often claim is possible) while others find that their baby cannot cope with an irregular 'let's see what we feel like' approach.

This 'irregular' approach is called demand-feeding, and means offering the baby milk every time he seems hungry. It often sorts itself out into a fairly predictable pattern, although not necessarily one of regular three- or four-hour intervals. If you have been hoping for a steady pattern around which you can plan your life, you may feel frustrated. But demand-feeding does not always have to be one-sided. You can make demands too, although perhaps it is more appropriate to think of it as a bit of give and take. For example, if breast-feeding is more of a duty than a pleasure, consider making one feed each day a bottle-feed of expressed breast milk or formula milk. The bottle can be given to the baby by someone else so that you can have some time to yourself.

However much you long for the predictability of feeds at precise times, you should also think of the possible disadvantages. Your life may not be so predictable once you start to get out and about more, and at times it may be more convenient for you to give your baby a feed earlier than usual rather than feel compelled to wait until the set time so that you do not upset his routine.

You may find that you are demand-feeding your baby because he has got used to frequent, small feeds. You may have stuck too rigidly to the 'ten minutes for each breast' guideline when, in fact, your milk takes longer to come in, or your circumstances may have been such that you have never had time to sit still for long enough to give him a full feed. (Some babies can take a whole feed in only a few minutes, but this usually happens when they are older and have developed a more efficient suck.) For example, if the birth coincided with moving house, you may have been continually distracted by getting the new home sorted out. You may have other children, too. Mothers with two or three other children sometimes find that their day is so interrupted with other demands that they never have time to give the baby more than half a feed at a time, so he ends up having twice as many feeds as planned.

Making the feeds more regular is a problem you can sort out only by setting times during the day when you insist that no one interrupts you except for a real emergency. Then you can sit down and give yourself and the baby time for a good feed. By allowing more time for him to feed, you help your baby to build up his appetite so that he gradually takes larger feeds.

Feeds do not have to be at four-hour intervals, as is often suggested. Just as older children can fit in three meals and a couple of snacks in eight to ten hours of the day, so some babies prefer to get most of what they need to eat during a similar period in the evening and at night when there are fewer distractions. Think of your baby needing the equivalent of about 1 litre (2 pt) of milk a day. At some feeds he may drink as much as 285 ml (½ pt) and at others only a small cupful. In this way feeds can resemble meals and snacks. If you find he is getting hungry before a time when you know you can concentrate on giving him a meal-sized feed, then you can offer him a quick snack-feed to keep him going until later. There is a limit to how often you can play this trick, as a hungry baby may get very upset if he cannot take his fill and be too tired by the time you are ready.

Feeds will also be less of a problem if you can keep everything you need in one place and always feed the baby there. If this isn't possible, it will save you some interruptions if you have a basket packed with nappies, tissues, something for you to drink, books for the toddler and so on, which you can pick up and take with you whenever you need to feed.

Bottle-feeding positively

However they are fed, babies can be a lot of hard work, and there is little point in adding problems to your labours by either breast-feeding reluctantly or bottle-feeding with a sense of guilt. More important than the method of feeding you choose is that you are happy and have a healthy, contented baby.

Bottle-fed babies are no more or less likely than breast-fed babies to cry, to demand feeding or to be sick (although there is some evidence that colic is more common in bottle-fed babies). How much you notice and are troubled by crying and upsets will depend considerably on how confident you feel. And if bottle-feeding gives you more confidence so that you are better able to cope, then that is probably the better way for you to feed your baby.

Think through your reasons for deciding to bottle-feed. If you have been upset trying to breast-feed, it may be only because you have had unrealistic expectations. Feeling guilty is demoralizing and unproductive. Instead, make a list of all the positive reasons for your decision and read them from time to time to reassure yourself.

If you wanted to breast-feed but circumstances have obliged you to bottle-feed, your baby may accept the breast as a comforter between feeds.

Changing from breast to bottle

If you have been breast-feeding and decide to change to the bottle, you will need to do it over a period of a couple of weeks. Your breasts may become engorged at first – probably because the relief of having reached a decision makes you more relaxed so that the let-down reflex is stimulated and you produce more milk. Start by dropping one breast-feed a day – the one that has the least milk – and substituting a bottle of formula milk. After a couple of days drop another feed, and continue in this way until you are down to just one feed, which you may like to continue as a comfort feed until your baby has lost interest.

Difficulties with bottle-feeding

If the baby is frequently sick after feeds or develops irritating rashes, you should see your doctor or health visitor before changing to another brand of formula. If the milk is disagreeing with the baby, your doctor needs to know. If the milk is not the cause of the problem, the health visitor may suggest a different way of managing the feed, such as a change in the size of the teat hole or the amount of the feed.

However you feed your baby, make the most of it and don't be hurried into weaning in order to end what may have seemed an unsatisfactory beginning.

Chapter 3
From three to six months

Current medical opinion in Britain is that babies should start eating solid foods between three and eight months of age. In some parts of the world weaning does not begin until the baby is about twelve months old, and then it is done rapidly. The age at which babies are started on solids varies not only from country to country, but also from one generation to another. In Britain alone it has been recommended at different times during the course of this century, and by different experts, that babies should start solids as early as one or two weeks of age, by six months, and not before nine months. The medical authorities who made these recommendations no doubt all did so in good faith and with good reason. However, advice that may suit a large number of babies will not suit all babies or their mothers.

Patterns of development

We have seen that new-born babies have reflexes that make them suck when stimulated and swallow any substance that comes in contact with the back of the tongue. A baby in the early weeks of life has difficulty taking food from a spoon because he is born with another reflex that causes him to push out with his tongue anything placed at the front of his mouth.

At three to four months all these automatic reflexes are weaker. By this age a baby has not only learnt to recognize the nipple or teat and open his mouth in readiness for it, but will also be eager and excited when he sees the breast or bottle, even licking his lips in anticipation. The reflex that causes him to push out food with his tongue is getting weaker and, the weaker the reflex, the easier it is for him to take food from a spoon. At about this age a baby begins to reach out for objects, though he will not yet be able to hold them unless they come within easy reach of his hands. Anything that is placed in his hands he will soon put in his mouth.

By five months a baby has gained full head control, which means he can turn his head away when he has had enough to eat. He may also try to grasp food from a plate if it comes within his reach. By six months he is capable of reaching out for food, grasping it and putting it in his mouth. He is also beginning to acquire the ability to move his jaw round and round – the movement that makes chewing possible. If bottle-fed, he may want to hold the bottle and may even insist on holding the spoon that feeds him. For the first six months a baby is content to be fed, but after this he will begin to want to have a hand in feeding himself.

Although a baby may be able to take food from a spoon somewhere between twelve and twenty weeks, do not expect him to rely on foods other than milk much before six months.

Does it matter how early solids are introduced? It is perfectly possible to make a baby of only one or two weeks of age swallow 'solid' food if it is put in a bottle and the teat hole enlarged. However, not only is this the same as force-feeding, but it also can be highly dangerous. It alters the nutritional balance of the baby's food supply, which strains his immature digestive system and kidneys. An over-concentrated feed also puts the baby at risk of dehydration. The practice in the past of giving very young babies bottle-feeds thickened with cereals is thought to have been a factor in the increase of coeliac disease – a disease in which the intestines are severely irritated by gluten, the protein in wheat.

Research into allergies also suggests that some babies – particularly those with a family history of allergies – are more at risk of developing allergies if their immature digestive systems are exposed to components in food that are different from those in breast milk. Medical experts generally advise that babies at high risk of developing allergies should be breast-fed exclusively for at least four months, and preferably six. Despite their apparent commonness and the considerable interest they excite, allergies affect only a minority of children, and there is little medical evidence that solids given as young as three months are likely to harm the health of most babies. (See Chapter 10.)

A baby is judged to be ready for weaning in two ways. He is physiologically ready to start solids when his digestive and immune systems are sufficiently developed to cope with foods other than milk. The average baby's digestive and immune systems are sufficiently mature between three and six months of age, but sometimes a little younger, or a little older in the case of babies with a family history of allergies.

A baby is developmentally ready for solids when he starts to explore objects with his mouth; takes an interest in what other people are eating, even trying to grab some for himself; and when the reflex that causes him to push food away with his tongue is sufficiently weakened so that he is able to keep thickish food like soups and paps in his mouth. This stage is usually entered between four and six months, though some babies will be ready a little younger and some a little older.

Problems with feeding

Establishing a regular pattern

Although demanding frequent feeds in practically no predictable pattern is perfectly normal behaviour in the case of tiny babies (see pp. 12–13), you may find it less acceptable as your baby grows older.

By about three months of age most babies are able to wait a bit for food and can take larger feeds. They are, therefore, at an age when they can be persuaded to have a more predictable pattern of feeding if they have not already developed one for themselves. There may, of course, still be days when your baby is a bit off-colour, out of sorts or going through a growth spurt and feeding becomes frequent and erratic. However, if in general your baby does not have a regular feeding routine at this age, and you find such irregularity or unpredictability difficult to cope with, try to introduce some kind of pattern into your day and the baby's.

Rather than setting times at which feeds should occur, you may find it easier to arrange a regular sequence of events around which feeds have to be fitted. For example, you can plan the baby's day so that it always includes getting up at a regular time, then getting dressed, an outing in the pram to the shops, a visit to someone else's house, a bath, playing with Dad in the evening and going to bed with a nursery rhyme. Babies with older siblings often develop a routine more quickly and easily than first babies because they have to fit in with the older children's very set pattern of life, including, perhaps, nursery school, meal times, television times and nap times.

Starting solids is another way in which a pattern is imposed on a baby. Dividing them into breakfast, midday and tea meals is a familiar routine that you may find easy to identify with and which can help establish a regular pattern.

Not enough milk

For six months – and sometimes a lot longer – breast or formula milk is able to supply all an infant's nutritional needs, provided the quantity is sufficient. (The exception to this is a baby who has never really thrived on milk, possibly because of a mild intolerance to cow's milk protein.) If he can take enough milk during the day to satisfy his appetite, by about three months the baby is able to drop one night feed, although the one he may prefer to do without could be the feed in the late evening rather than the middle of the night! Waking in the night is common during infancy. It is not necessarily a sign of hunger, and sometimes the baby may be satisfied just to suck.

Some babies – particularly large ones – need much more milk than others, and instead of cutting out a feed by three months, they may be asking for an extra one. If your baby is hungry, more milk will satisfy him and, provided he gets enough, he will thrive. However, not all mothers are prepared to go back to more frequent feeding, particularly if it means more disturbed nights. Some breast-feeding mothers find that, however much more rest or food they take, after three months they cannot increase their milk supply any more. There are two alternatives: to give the baby one or two complementary bottle-feeds or to start him on solids, although it may take a month or so before he is taking sufficient solids to make any real impact on his appetite. If solids do seem to make a breast-fed baby more settled, then the chances are he is getting more milk from you because you have begun to relax – and so produce more

milk – once he is no longer solely dependent on you for
his food. This is not unlike the sudden increase in the
milk flow experienced by some mothers once they have
decided to go over to bottle-feeding because breast-
feeding is too difficult.

Introducing the bottle

Giving the bottle as well as the breast requires a delicate
balance: you have to bottle-feed sufficiently frequently
so that the baby gets used to it, but not so often that
either your breast milk diminishes because of a slacken-
ing in demand or the baby develops a marked preference
for the bottle. A bottle is much less work for a baby;
some babies prefer an easy life even if it does mean a
rubber teat whereas others definitely prefer the smell
and feel of the breast.

On the whole, new-born babies will take either the
breast or the bottle with equal ease, but the older
the baby is, the harder it can be to get him to accept the
bottle. If it is important that your baby is able to accept a
bottle as well as the breast, it is probably best to start
giving him a bottle of expressed breast milk every few
days from about four to six weeks.

In the case of an older baby you may have to introduce
the bottle with a little subterfuge. You can start by
dipping the teat in a little expressed breast milk and
letting him lick it off the outside. It may also help if your
partner introduces the bottle so that the baby is not
distracted by the smell and feel of you. Once he seems
quite happy with this new toy, you can start him on
small amounts of milk about an hour before he is likely
to need a feed so that he is not desperate with hunger. If
he is resistant, it may help to give him a dummy or an
empty bottle as a toy to hold and put in his mouth. You

will need to offer it each day until he gradually gets accustomed to it. Once he seems happy to taste a dummy, you can start him on the bottle again. Don't try to force the bottle into his mouth: you will only teach him to fight harder. But if a breast-fed baby has no choice, however much resistance he may put up, eventually he will feed from the bottle – though it may mean a distressing and very hungry twenty-four hours!

Successful weaning

Babies do not need to start solids before six months at the earliest if they have an adequate supply of milk. However, most mothers in Britain are eager to wean their babies as soon as they can without incurring the disapproval of other mothers or the medical profession. The currently 'approved' age is three to four months. Mothers who do not start weaning their babies at this age often report that they feel under pressure from society and the health care professions to do so, and the longer they leave it, the 'odder' they are made to feel.

At one time it was thought that babies needed more of certain nutrients, particularly iron, by the age of six months. Research has shown that iron is supplied in breast milk, and it is added to formula milk. If a baby is having five or six feeds of breast or formula milk a day, he should be getting sufficient iron and vitamins, and there is no need to hurry him on to solids.

Whatever age you start to wean your baby, the key to success is to follow *his* pace, one step at a time, and ignore how quickly other babies are supposedly taking to solids. The stage of development your baby is at can make a considerable difference to the ease with which he takes to solids. For example, at three months a baby can be introduced to solids only if some food is put in his mouth, whereas at six months he may initiate the weaning process by grabbing something off his mother's plate and putting it in his mouth. At three months a baby licks his lips when he recognizes food – he expects to enjoy his meal – whereas at six months he may have developed certain discriminating powers and can show he is more interested in some foods than others. A three-month-old baby may retch or gag in response to a physical stimulus, such as too much food in his mouth or a spoon touching the back of his tongue, but at six months he may gag simply as the result of an alarmed expression on his mother's face. At three months he cannot try to feed himself, but at six months he may make it very clear that he will not eat unless he is allowed to try to feed himself. A three-month-old baby has to have all his food puréed, but at six months he is able to chew on soft pieces of food like rusks, banana or cooked vegetables.

When you start to give your baby solids, think of the first tastes as a bit of fun and do not expect him to replace any milk in his diet. Setting a date by which you expect your baby to be eating a meal-sized portion of food or have eaten enough to drop a feed can slow down the process, as he will probably sense you are trying to hurry him. If he is still enjoying sucking, he may be all the more reluctant to give up the bottle or breast. If there is a date by which you have to have dropped one or two breast-feeds – for example, if someone else is going to be looking after your child – then it is better to spend more time encouraging a young baby to take milk from a bottle. That way, if he has a spell when he doesn't want solids, you will know that he can be fed and comforted by sucking from a bottle if you can't be with him.

Chapter 4
From six to twelve months

Patterns of development

If a baby has started solids at four months or a bit earlier, by six months he will probably be on three proper meals and have dropped one or two milk feeds during the day.

At around six to eight months a baby is beginning to become aware that he can do some things for himself. By this age he is likely to have sufficient head control to be able to turn his head away to show that he has eaten enough. He may want to hold the bottle or spoon that feeds him or may try to grab any object or food that comes within his reach. Once anything is in his hands, he will most likely take it to his mouth, occasionally examining an object by passing it from one hand to the other.

A baby likes to explore different textures in his mouth and will be interested in the thickness of cereal, the slipperiness of mashed banana, the crisp then soggy texture of a rusk, the lumpiness of a few rice grains and so on. He will probably begin to show likes and dislikes of food, and may begin to prefer foods that are brightly coloured or have an interesting shape. Rusks, soft pieces of fruit and vegetables are particularly attractive – they have definite shapes, and they are things he can hold and feed to himself.

At this age a baby is also becoming increasingly aware of the different tones in his mother's voice. He can tell when she is cross, anxious, happy or alarmed and he may respond in a similar fashion. If, for example, a mother is anxious about what her baby is eating, he may become anxious too, and if his mother shows alarm, it can trigger off his gag reflex.

His ability to take solids now improves and he will take food from the spoon more cleanly, without much of it oozing out of the corners of his mouth. However, being competent at spoon-feeding does not mean that his eating will be clean and tidy. He will want to explore his food with his hands by, for example, splashing his hands in his bowl, trying to pick up a pea, watching what happens when he squeezes porridge through his fingers – and in the middle of all this he will find that he really must scratch behind his ear! Of course, not all babies are alike. Just as some like cuddly toys and some don't, so some babies find food particularly fascinating while others are content just to eat rather than play with it.

As a baby gets older, his eating skills and discrimination improve. He gets better at picking up small objects like a kernel of sweet corn or a bean, and he begins to drink more than a few sips from a beaker or cup. He begins to chew more efficiently and will discover how to bite so that he can manage sandwiches, biscuits and large chunks of fruit. He will want to feed himself more, trying to grasp the spoon when it comes near his mouth. If he sees a food he likes, he will get excited, and if he sees something he doesn't like, he will protest by throwing his body back and stiffening with resistance. He also learns to understand the meaning of 'no' – though that does not mean he will obey it.

Common weaning problems

Although the majority of children are weaned at some stage during the first year, there is no particular age at

which it is best to start. Whenever you start, the introduction of solids will be easier if you are confident that
your baby is thriving on breast or formula milk. However, once a baby is on solids, progress isn't always
smooth and steady. Some babies go one step back before
they go two steps forward. For example, your baby may
have been happily taking solids before his milk feed, and
then suddenly start to fret and want his milk first. This
is not unusual and if you play along for a week or two
you should be able to help him regain his confidence. It's
worth remembering that most parents who worry about
their babies not eating have babies that are well grown
and even fat – though it can be hard to realize until you
are able to look back at old baby photos. If your baby is
growing, he is not undernourished.

Refuses to start solids

A young baby – one who is less than six or even eight
months old – may simply not be ready to start solids. He
may still have a highly developed tongue thrust or bite
reflex, which makes it difficult for him to take food from
a spoon. These reflexes will weaken with time. Most
babies under six months also have a strong sucking urge,
and if your baby feels solids are depriving him of some of
his much-loved sucking time, he may resist. If he does
not seem interested in starting solids, forget about it for
a couple of weeks and then try again.

If you have been trying to give your baby solids every
couple of days over several weeks and he has proved
resistant, he may have become anxious about feeding,
and be protesting more strongly at each attempt. The
reason may be not so much that he dislikes solids –
although he may soon learn to do so if they always signal
a battle – as that he very much prefers the breast or

bottle. A young baby may be easier to wean, therefore, if
he is allowed to have half of his milk feed first.

If your baby has become very suspicious of the spoon,
he may be happier to start solids when he can take the
initiative. If he is over six months, you can sit him on
your lap while you eat. His natural curiosity will make
him want to investigate your plate – so don't try this
when you are eating hot food. A breakfast meal of cereal
and toast or a sandwich are ideal and the ingredients are
suitable for a baby this age. Although he may try to taste
some food, don't be dismayed if he only plays with it.
The object of the exercise is to kindle his interest in
solids, whether that means poking his finger in it and
squashing it a bit, or simply watching you eating. And if
his 'play' looks like proving too messy, it will be a new
experience for him to have you take food away rather
than try to push it into his mouth! You could also place
little pieces of cooked vegetables, soft fruits or a rusk in
a bowl or on the tray of his high chair for him to
investigate.

Allowing the older baby to find out about solids for
himself will please him because it is an opportunity for
him to exert his independence and will enable him to
get used to the idea of foods other than milk at his own
pace.

While you are waiting for his interest in solids to
develop, try to get his milk feeds into a regular pattern, if
they are not already, so that you can get him used to
breakfast, lunch and tea mealtimes.

Still wants frequent milk feeds

Erratic, frequent feeds are more likely in a breast-fed
than a bottle-fed baby, as it is more difficult for a mother
to distinguish between full feeds and comfort sucks

when breast-feeding. By the time a baby is six months old – and often well before this – it is possible for him to get most of a feed within a few minutes, so that short comfort sucks and feeds can be much the same length of time.

To reduce the frequency of feeds, start to think of breast-feeding primarily as a way of providing food rather than comfort. Give your baby all the time he wants when it is a feed, but reduce sucking at the breast between feeds. He is old enough to form attachments to other comfort objects, so you can give him a particular toy or piece of cloth to cuddle when he is fretful or just cuddle him without giving him the breast. If he still has a strong desire to suck and does not already take a bottle, encourage him to take water or juice from a bottle rather than breast-feed. Discourage him from falling asleep on the breast or bottle; if he associates falling asleep with the comfort of the nipple, he may wake in the night and have difficulty getting back to sleep without the help of a bit of sucking.

Alternatively, you may prefer to continue with the breast as a comforter between feeds while getting the baby to use a spoon and a beaker at meals. If so, be prepared for your baby to go on wanting the breast for some time, particularly if he has no substitute comfort objects. Although many babies naturally tire of the breast or bottle by about twelve months, some do not. Encourage your baby to derive comfort from another object if only to give yourself some peace of mind should you ever be ill or have to leave him in someone else's care for a while.

If your baby has a persistent need to suck and seems to be especially fretful or suffer from lots of colds and snuffles, it may be a sign that he is unwell, and you should consult your doctor or health visitor. Sick babies will often want more comfort sucking than usual: a bit of cosseting and extra mothering is always welcome during illness, even when one is an adult.

Won't drop any milk feeds or wants to restart them

Sometimes, although a baby seems to be taking to solids well, he may refuse to drop any of the accompanying breast- or bottle-feeds, or suddenly refuse all solids and go back to full breast- or bottle-feeding. In this case, particularly if he wants to go back to all milk feeds, a baby does enjoy solids, but is not sure he is ready to be weaned off the breast or bottle.

Rather than persisting with trying to get your baby to drop a feed, let him do as he wants for a week or two and then try again to get him to drop a feed or to start solids. If he feels he is no longer being pushed into giving up his beloved bottle or breast, he should relax and be prepared to rely less on milk.

Won't give up night feeds

Some babies progress well with weaning during the day – happy to take solids and drinks from a cup or beaker with a milk feed in the morning and/or one at bedtime – but seem to want several feeds during the night, almost returning to their new-born habits! Night waking is very common in babies and young children, and can start at any time for no obvious reason. In older babies it is often blamed on teething, and this may indeed be the problem if one of the baby's cheeks is red and he is dribbling more than usual. If he is not teething and seems to want only a bit of comfort sucking rather than being ravenous for a feed, he may want to be assured that the breast or bottle, which is being given less often during the day, is still there when he wants it. However well a baby takes to solids it is perfectly natural for him to still want to have his sucking urge satisfied.

Before you try to stop night feeds you need to work out exactly what you feel about them. If you too are missing that special contact and feel a bit reluctant about your baby growing up so fast, you may decide that the pleasure of being together, especially if it is peaceful, outweighs the discomfort of lost sleep.

Although one or two night feeds can be soothing for both of you, if he seems to want to suck more frequently or be developing a habit, you may find it more difficult to cope. If you start to resent night feeds, work out how you are going to handle the situation *before* you put your baby to bed. Waking is not so much the problem as the fact that the baby is unable to settle himself back to sleep without some assistance. Giving him a drink of water from a bottle or stroking him while he is lying in his cot can help break the habit – he knows you are there but is not fully woken by being lifted. If this does not work, you may decide to limit him to a set number of feeds during the night (if he wakes a lot) and the rest of the time either lift him for a cuddle or leave him in his cot, touching and talking to him or behaving in much the same way as when he needs comfort during the day.

Night waking can often be cured if someone else is able to attend the baby during the night. Many a mother who has had to leave her baby in someone else's care for a few nights, perhaps because she was ill, found that the baby soon learnt to go back to sleep without her presence. If you want to try this procedure, you and your husband might agree that he will sleep in the baby's room for a couple of nights. For this approach to have any chance of success, your husband has to be allowed to be in complete charge, without any interference from you.

Once your baby has had his last breast-feed, you may feel a bit upset. If you are worried that any subsequent fretfulness is caused by his missing the breast, you can reassure yourself by offering it to him again after about a week. You will almost certainly find that he looks quite puzzled, as if he is wondering what on earth you expect him to do with it!

Won't drink from beaker or cup

For the first six months, most babies still have a strong urge to suck, which a beaker or a cup does not satisfy. A baby who has a strong suck can splutter and choke on a beaker because he has drawn too much liquid at once. As he gets older, his sucking urge will decrease, and he may find it easier to take liquid from a cup than a beaker. If you start with a small cup, about the size of an egg cup, there will be less problem of the liquid coming out fast. A small cup also enables the baby to have the reassurance of seeing you over the rim. If you think it is the taste of water or juice he does not like, then give him some of his usual milk to drink. In the meantime let him familiarize himself with the cup or beaker by playing with it. Babies who are not keen on cups or the taste of water will often learn to drink water out of cups or other vessels – such as toy boats – while playing in the bath. If you don't like the idea of your baby drinking bath water, give him opportunities to play with a few plastic mugs and a large bowl of clean water. When he has acquired the skill of drinking from a beaker or cup, you can confidently offer him drinks from it at one and then two meals instead of always feeling obliged to offer him the breast or bottle.

Won't drink or refuses milk

A baby who refuses drinks is usually getting enough liquid from his food and milk. Provided he continues to produce wet nappies at every change time, he is not dehydrated.

When a baby tires of the breast or bottle, he will sometimes decline milk altogether, probably because he liked it only while he enjoyed sucking. If you have always been led to believe that children need milk in order to stay healthy, you may find it worrying if he refuses to drink any. Milk has been particularly valued because it is one of the few rich sources of calcium and because it is often drunk in large quantities. But there are many parts of the world where children and adults do not drink milk and yet do not suffer calcium deficiency. Calcium, like iron, is a nutrient that the body can absorb in larger proportions when the amount in the diet is small. Although milk is a nutritionally valuable food, it is not the only one. Baked beans and bread are good all-rounders too. In terms of satisfying his calorie requirements, if a child drinks little but satisfies his appetite in other ways, his health will not suffer.

A baby who does not like drinking milk will often take it in other forms, for example, in yoghurt, custard, as cheese or in proprietary baby foods. Although it is highly unlikely that your baby will be at any risk of calcium deficiency, you can feed him baby cereals or foods that have had calcium added (see the labels on the packets) if it will reassure you.

Small appetite

There are a number of reasons why your baby's appetite may diminish at this age. In the first six months of his life a baby gains two-thirds of the weight he will put on in the whole of the first year. After six months the rate at which he gains weight will be a bit slower and this may make it seem as if he is losing his appetite. He also may not be particularly hungry if he is not very active because he has not yet learnt to crawl. He may be fighting the spoon because he wants to feed himself – and it can be a disconcerting sight to see a six- or seven-month-old baby firmly closing his lips for this reason! You may be overestimating how much he needs or underestimating how much milk, or even biscuits or rusks, he is consuming. He may need longer gaps between meals, and his need for play and sleep can be more powerful than his desire for food.

If your baby is bright-eyed, generally interested in what is going on and growing in length, then it is very unlikely that he is ill. His appetite may improve when he becomes more mobile, though some babies simply become much thinner, because they are still growing in length without any noticeable improvement in appetite. He may also prefer more opportunity to feed himself. You could try giving him a spoon with some food on it or giving him a spoon and a bowl containing a small portion of food. While he is trying to work out the mechanics of getting a spoon into his bowl and from there into his mouth, he may be willing for you to feed him, though it can be a slow process. If hunger for your own meal is making you irritable, then eat first and leave him to nibble a few cubes of vegetables until it is his turn.

You could try lengthening the time between his meals, but then beware of giving him something to eat in the intervals. Biscuits and rusks between meals can be a common cause of eating problems. They are items a baby is often given when he is grizzly to keep him quiet, which teaches him to regard them as a source of comfort. They are foods he is allowed to hold himself, which makes them more desirable than foods he has to be fed. They usually have a strong taste, either sweet or salty, for which he can easily acquire a liking. He can eat them as slowly as he likes without being chivvied about dawdling, and if he is allowed to eat them sitting on the floor with his toys, they will seem much more fun than the food for which he is made to sit in a high chair. For all these reasons, avoid biscuits as much as possible, particularly if he has a small appetite.

If your baby really is not interested in his food, he will come to no harm if he misses a meal from time to time. However, if he is a persistently small eater, it would be a wise precaution to give him the breast or a modified milk formula, which is fortified with extra vitamins and minerals, rather than plain cow's milk.

Retching

A baby may retch or gag when he has too much food in his mouth, or if the food is too thick or he has had enough and does not want any more. Your baby may have a particularly strong gag reflex, which is usually far more alarming for you than for him. If he has had enough and you try to make him take 'just one more spoonful', he may simply vomit the whole lot back.

Chapter 5
The toddler

After the first birthday a baby's growth slows down considerably, and many toddlers need less food and so eat less. Indeed, if a child were to continue growing at the rate shown in his first year, he would be 29 metres (96 ft) tall and weigh 200 tonnes by his tenth birthday. Losing his appetite or developing fads about which foods he will and will not eat is common between twelve months and four and a half years, and can be described almost as normal behaviour.

Whatever the size of his appetite, your toddler may have a pot-belly and a chubby face. Toddlers, like new-born babies, vary enormously in size, and chubby toddlers may eat the same amount as, or even less than, children of a more petite build. From the age of about three he should gradually thin down and his limbs will lengthen.

Patterns of development

During toddlerhood a child is acquiring and refining a number of physical skills, such as walking, running and jumping, and is becoming able to understand more and work things out. He begins to assert his independence, which can be truly thrilling for him, but may make your heart sink several times a day as he explores and tries out his new-found freedom.

The problems that so often arise at this age are not all a conflict between a parent and child, for the child is often having battles with himself. A toddler can find life very frustrating, for example, because his physical and mental skills do not develop at the same rate and he cannot always get his body to do what his mind wants. And although he will probably revel in his new skills and his increasing ability to do things for himself, he may also get a bit frightened by this independence from time to time. This is likely to make him cling to his comforters, occasionally reverting to more babyish habits in his need for reassurance.

The second twelve months

At about twelve months your baby may be trying to feed himself with a spoon, although, because he has only a limited wrist action at this age, he will find it difficult and may then insist on using his fingers or thrust the bowl out of the way. He can hold his cup or beaker if it is handed to him, but probably is not yet able to pick it up for himself. He may constantly be throwing things on to the floor, including his beaker or cup, food, spoon – and even his bowl. He likes having these objects handed back to him and may get cross if you don't scrape his food off the floor and return it to him like any other toy! He may discover the art of spitting out food, which will give rise to great glee and encouragement from an older child. He will begin to shake his head or say 'no', though at first more to see how you react than because he means it. He is also good at pointing to objects he wants – like the biscuit tin.

These skills give your child new ways of communicating with you, and the more he can direct your attention, the more pleased he will be. If throwing down his spoon every few seconds, blowing raspberries with his custard or shaking his head makes you react in a particular way, he may be eager to repeat the exercise in order to get the same response. At first you might find these gestures, including saying no, charming, but he soon will become more assertive and insistent; then when he says no, you may find yourself locked in a battle of wills. Unfortunately for parents, the toddler almost invariably wins such battles, as it is easy – particularly if the dispute is over something you consider important – for your normal ability to handle difficulties to become clouded by emotions in your natural concern for your infant's well-being.

At fifteen months an infant is more skilled at licking food off a spoon, although he still has difficulty keeping it the right way up. He is able to chew better, but it will still be several months before he is fully competent. He can make his wants for food better understood, as he can point more exactly and will emphasize it by 'talking' and bouncing up and down.

He is likely to be very restless and to want to be constantly on the move. Like many toddlers, he may consider finding his feet – literally – and finding ways to satisfy his curiosity more exciting than eating, which may make him resistant to being put in a high chair and having a harness put on to prevent him falling out. Meals can become a real bore from his point of view if he sees them as always restricting his freedom. He is, however, very easily distracted, and you may be able to divert his attention by putting a few crumbs of food or grains of cooked rice on his tray so that he can practise picking up tiny objects. Although this activity cannot be counted on for more than a few seconds, it will probably give you enough time to get him seated and harnessed.

At eighteen months your baby may be able to manage a spoon without spilling much, but feeding will still be fairly messy. He will enjoy activities like building towers with his toys, putting objects in and taking them out of containers, and playing with water. For a child, especially one who is not particularly hungry, food may be another kind of toy to be played with. Just as he likes to take things to bits to see how they 'work', he may want to pull his food apart, watch what happens when it is squashed and then pile it all up again. Although this can make meals slow as well as messy, not allowing him to play with his food in this way won't necessarily speed up his eating.

From two to three years

By about the age of two years your child will probably be able to feed himself competently, although he will still be slow and untidy. Now that he has proved he can do it himself, he may be happy to let – and even want – you to spoon-feed him from time to time. Feeding him may speed up meals, but you may have to pay the price of making him lazy about feeding himself.

As he discovers the routines that govern everyday activities, he may start to develop his own rituals, such as refusing to eat a biscuit if it is broken, demanding a clean knife to spread his jam with or insisting that you do not allow any one food to touch another on his plate – even though he may then mix them together himself. Such rules, which a child cannot explain in words, can be baffling to an adult, who regards them from a very different point of view. Your toddler may want the crusts cut off his bread not because he finds them hard to chew, but, probably, because he likes the way his sandwiches look without them. And because he cannot explain what he wants, he may simply refuse to eat until he is offered something in a form he considers acceptable.

At this age a child has no sense of time apart from the

present. He can think only of his immediate wants and needs, and is not able to plan ahead. An adult may eat when she is not particularly hungry in order not to get hungry before the next meal is due, but a toddler won't understand that he may get hungry later if he doesn't eat now. Similarly, when he is hungry, your child will want food immediately, but if a meal is ready and he has found a new toy, he may be unable to concentrate on eating until he has finished playing and will need a few reminders that playtime is coming to an end.

At two he will be acquiring yet more skills, which might include drinking through a straw and unscrewing the top of a bottle. This is the age when a child – boy or girl – wants to imitate domestic activities and will be eager to 'help' you with the shopping, cooking, washing-up and feeding a doll (or a younger brother or sister!). Although he may be happy to play with a toy kitchen and tea set, he will probably prefer the real thing and insist on pouring his drink or stirring his food himself. If thwarted, your child may become extremely rebellious and throw a tantrum. You may still be able to distract him fairly easily, as he is intensely curious. However, avoid using food, particularly biscuits and sweets, to divert and calm him now. If you regularly use food as a pacifier your child may learn to throw tantrums to get a biscuit he would otherwise be refused.

Between eighteen months and three years a child is particularly eager to exert his will, especially over other members of the family. He will leap with alacrity on any situation where he feels he can take control, especially if he is lively and strong-willed. At this age the commonest problem areas are eating, sleeping, using the potty and throwing tantrums because a child soon discovers that no one can force him to eat, sleep, use the potty or be quiet if he chooses not to.

Simple solutions to everyday problems

A toddler learning to feed himself with a spoon is often messy and awkward. A clean plastic cloth under the high chair will protect the floor and enable you to rescue some of the food. A supply of spoons will prevent you from having to retrieve each one as it is thrown. It may help if you give your child only one or two pieces of finger food at a time or put only a tiny portion in his bowl to which you can add when necessary.

You can give an outlet to his desire for independence by letting him choose his food from a serving dish. This does not mean he is given a choice of *what* to eat, but that he can choose the order and quantity put in his bowl.

If his bowl is in continual danger of being thrown on the floor, try one with a suction pad on the base, a heavy pottery bowl, or a plastic bowl sold for pets which has sloping sides and is difficult to tip over.

If he tends to get his clothes in a mess, roll up his sleeves as well as giving him a long-sleeved bib. If he still manages to get food under his bib and down his clothes, you can dress him in a nylon all-in-one showerproof outfit, worn back to front so that the zip does not get gummed up with food. Coping with mess in this way may be more satisfactory than trying to make your baby eat tidily, particularly if, as a result, he feels you are trying to thwart his efforts to feed himself.

Common eating problems

A small appetite

Probably the commonest eating problem in this age group is a small appetite. The first thing to understand is that a small appetite can be quite normal at this age and need not indicate anything unfavourable about your child's physical health or emotional well-being. Health professionals frequently try to reassure mothers by telling them that no healthy child will let itself starve, though one well-known paediatrician has added the rider 'unless force-fed'.[1]

There are several reasons why a child may eat little. It is easy to overestimate how much a toddler needs as well as to underestimate how much he is already eating. For example, a child who drinks several glasses of milk and undiluted fruit juice a day will be obtaining a sizeable proportion of calories from these drinks alone, but because they are drinks you may not think of them as foods when you are estimating how much he is eating.

A toddler's appetite can vary enormously from one meal to the next, just like an adult's, and your child may eat well on one day and then eat very little for the next two or three days. He has not yet learnt the social habit of eating and, unlike an adult, if he is not hungry, he simply won't eat. Eating only when hungry rather than when the time or occasion demands can be a virtue worth preserving in a society where so many adults have weight problems. Young children are usually much more interested in exercise than food whereas their parents are often the opposite.

A toddler may eat little because he has a small build. Relatively little food energy, measured in calories,[2] is needed for growth after the first few months of life, only

[1] Ronald S. Illingworth, *The Normal Child*, 7th edn, Edinburgh, Churchill Livingstone, 1979.
[2] Calories are tiny units, and what most people refer to as a calorie is really 1,000 calories, or a kilocalorie. However, in everyday usage the prefix 'kilo' is usually omitted.

about 5 kilocalories for each gramme of weight gained, which is roughly 37 calories a day for a child in its second year. Most of the calories a child eats are spent on just keeping the body's metabolism working. Although acute and chronic ill-health can affect the appetite, a previously well-nourished child will also have built up good supplies of nutrients that can be drawn upon over many months if necessary. The under-fives have a remarkable capacity to compensate later for the growth they may seem to be missing out on now. If you think back to your own childhood, you may be able to remember children who seemed small for their age at primary school but at least of average height when they were at secondary school.

Sometimes a child refuses food because he has learnt to associate meal times with misery. Much of the pleasure may have gone out of eating if he has been coerced to eat tidily before he is ready, if he has not been allowed to feed himself when he wanted to, or if he has been constantly coaxed to eat more than he wants. In these circumstances a poor appetite may become a habit rather than a passing phase.

Refusing food – or certain foods – is also an opportunity for a child to demonstrate his independence and to test how far he can usurp his parents' control over what he does. Having a toddler who seems set to defy you can be very embarrassing as well as hurtful and you may be very tempted to let him have his own way. But giving in to your child is not any better than always letting battles develop. A toddler who wants an opportunity to prove he is boss may feel just as thwarted if he meets no resistance as if he has to face enormous obstacles. A mother who tries to impose her will on her toddler and one who gives in to her toddler all the time are in fact both trying to force a child to eat. One mother does it by nagging and the other by coaxing. A child who is continually being made to eat 'just a few more spoonfuls' or is repeatedly given snacks or biscuits between meals because he hasn't eaten may soon find food a huge obstruction between himself and everything he wants to do. The chances are that if you are continually preoccupied with what your child has or has not eaten, he will feel similarly plagued by the tedium of eating, and the result will be a vicious circle.

A toddler's temperament can also affect how much he eats. A lively, energetic child will often eat *less* than a quiet child. Sitting down to eat is an activity that better suits a placid child than one who needs to be on the go all the time. It is known from studies on adults that some of the calories eaten are not used by the body. People vary considerably in the extent to which their bodies lose or store this surplus energy, and it is quite likely that toddlers vary in much the same way. The placid toddler who eats well but does not get fat may be wasting more energy than the active, energetic child who may eat little but uses the small amounts of energy he gets from food very efficiently.

If your child has a small appetite and you have reason to suspect his health is suffering, you should, of course, consult your doctor. You probably will be told there is nothing to worry about and that if you ignore the child's small appetite and, maybe, let him eat whatever he wants, the problem will eventually resolve itself. Such advice, although easy to give, is not always simple to follow without a bit more help, and it must not be taken too literally. After all, a child who is encouraged to eat *anything* he likes might end up living in a sweet shop!

It is important to make meals a pleasure. Food can give pleasure not simply because it fills an empty tummy, but also because it looks good, smells good and is eaten in a congenial atmosphere. A child may enjoy exploring the feel of food and take pleasure in the sight of an attractive dish without necessarily wanting to taste it. Giving him occasions when he can play with food allows him to explore food in his own way. The following suggestions may help you rekindle your child's interest in food, but don't expect an improvement in his appetite immediately.

1. Let him help you prepare food

An adult may prefer food that has been prepared for him, but a child is generally more interested if he has participated in preparing and serving the meal. He can play with pastry, wash vegetables, mix salads, fetch saucepans and empty frozen vegetables out of the packet ready for cooking. If he does not show much interest in such domestic activities, he will almost certainly enjoy playing with flour, sticking a (clean) finger in the butter or margarine, and making patterns or building towers with pieces of raw carrot or pasta shapes.

2. Put the food for a meal on a serving dish

Ask your toddler to point to what he wants and, if he can, help himself. If he chooses to start with, say, peas, put just a few on his plate, and do this with each food until he decides he has enough. When he finishes a first portion, ask him if he wants more; if he does not, don't press him. Both you and he will get more pleasure if he is allowed to start with a tiny helping and ask for more (or not, as the case may be) than if he eats only one teaspoonful from a much larger portion that is left on the plate.

Serving food in this way also enables a child to become familiar with new foods. In time he will want to taste some of the new foods he sees. Some he will like and some he won't. Provided no fuss is made, he will most likely try a new taste again a few days or weeks later when he has become used to seeing the food at fairly regular intervals.

3. Let him eat on his own

Most children from twelve months on can feed themselves, even if it does mean using their hands rather than a spoon. If your urge is to keep watching to see how much he is eating or to keep 'helping' him to get the food into his mouth, it may be better not to sit next to your child. Distance yourself as much as possible and leave him to explore his food in peace. Once it is clear he is not going to eat any more, remove the plate and, if appropriate, offer him something else.

4. Don't give him sweets

It is unwise to offer a child with a poor appetite sugary puddings or sweet snacks if there is a danger of them replacing more nourishing foods. Most children – including poor eaters – like sweet foods and often learn to refuse all other foods if they think they have a good chance of getting the sweet food they want. Instead of a prepared pudding, you can offer a piece of fruit, which is sweet but has the virtue of supplying some vitamins and minerals as well. A piece of bread may also be a welcome follow-on to an uneaten first course, as it is a nourishing, filling food and can be held in the hand with little mess.

5. Control between-meal snacks

Ideally there should be no eating between meals. A toddler, if given the choice, would usually prefer to eat between, rather than at, mealtimes because such snacks are usually something he is allowed to hold in his hand, eat where he wants and as slowly or as fast as he likes. If the food offered is chocolate or a biscuit, it is an added attraction. A child with a small appetite often doesn't have difficulty in clamouring for more biscuits or sweet drinks! It is not so much that eating between meals is undesirable as the kind of foods that tend to be offered then. If you feel it is too drastic a step to cut out between-meal snacks, give your child wholesome foods like cold vegetables or a chunk of bread.

Sometimes, of course, there is genuine hunger between meals. For example, a child who wants his breakfast at dawn cannot wait six hours or more until the midday meal. If your child needs shorter intervals between the times he eats, give him four or even five small meals a day. A dawn waker could be given an early breakfast of, for example, milk and bread-and-butter or a banana followed by a more conventional breakfast at a later time. A child who goes to bed late could be given a sandwich or a yoghurt for supper before bedtime. As always, you should give a child healthy foods rather than sweet or salty snack foods.

If biscuits and crisps are already part of your child's diet, rather than banning them, you could limit them to one meal a day. Making them part of a meal – on a plate and at table – often makes these foods slightly less attractive than when they are eaten between meals. Also if the child feels assured that he will be offered biscuits or crisps at some stage, he may gradually learn to demand them less.

6. Reduce his consumption of milk

A child with a small appetite may need to have his milk intake reduced if he regularly drinks more than 570 ml (1 pt) a day, as larger quantities of milk may take the edge off his appetite. One way to do this is to limit milk drinks to only one or two meals a day, but allow him to drink his fill at these times. Alternatively, you can put a limited amount in a jug and not refill it when it is empty. If you find it difficult to get your child to drink less milk, give him semi-skimmed or skimmed milk to see whether fewer calories from milk improve his appetite for other foods.

Large quantities of fruit juice can also have a dulling effect on a small appetite because of the calories supplied by the natural sugars in them (this also makes them bad for teeth if drunk frequently between meals). You can partially dilute fruit juice or try well-diluted fruit-flavoured drinks, which often have a more concentrated taste for fewer calories.

7. *Do not confuse encouraging your child to eat with disciplining him*

If discipline is what really concerns you, make a few rules that are not related to how much he eats. For example, at this age it is appropriate to insist that he sits down while he is eating and does not deliberately throw food around. You can also limit the amount of time he has a dish in front of him, and not allow him to watch television during mealtimes. Any rules you do make should, of course, be consistent with your general approach to handling his behaviour. Generally, the fewer rules you make, the better your chances of getting them followed.

8. *Don't discuss his eating habits in his hearing*

This is probably the hardest advice of all when a toddler needs to be kept so much in your sight. A child can understand far more than you might guess from the amount he talks, and knowing he is attracting attention in this way is likely to encourage the poor eating habits you are trying to overcome.

If you can teach yourself to defuse the emotional atmosphere surrounding mealtimes by paying less attention to what your child does or does not eat, his diet will gradually become less of an issue. If he continues to look healthy and well – and most children with poor appetites are usually flourishing in other ways – you can rest assured that he is eating enough to meet his needs.

Food fads

Although most toddlers tend to prefer familiar foods to unfamiliar ones, some children have such firm likes and dislikes that they eat only a very limited range of foods. Food fads can not only disrupt family meals – for example, if no one is served chicken because the toddler will not eat it – but also can become a serious social handicap if they continue after the child has started school. This problem is particularly likely to arise in a child who does not eat much and, in order to get him to eat, has been given only foods that he will eat. When this happens the toddler soon learns that he has the power to dictate what he is given, especially if he is regularly asked whether he would like to have a particular food for lunch or tea. Most canny toddlers when asked a question beginning 'Do you want . . . ?' will nearly always answer 'No' even before they have heard the full question!

Before you take any remedial action make a list of everything your toddler will eat and drink, however small the quantities. Include such information as whether he eats white as well as brown bread and cheese cooked as well as fresh. This list will be a useful reminder when you are planning what to give him to eat, and may also show you that he has a more varied diet than you think. If you find that there are one or two foods that he is consuming in large quantities, including milk (see pp. 47–8), restrict his intake of them to encourage him to develop an appetite for other foods. If he is particularly fussy about eating fruits or vegetables, consult your doctor about giving him vitamin drops to reassure yourself that he is not being deprived of essential nutrients.

If your child is used to being asked what he wants, offer him a choice of any two items on the list you have made. You can also allow him to choose having his potatoes or vegetables served first. If he wants to eat his pudding before his first course, no harm will be done if the pudding is a piece of fruit, which might just as well be eaten as a starter as a dessert. Letting him choose between foods you approve allows him to make a choice but at the same time prevents him from dictating what he will or will not eat at each meal. If he wants to change his mind, you should feel confident about being firm with him because you know it is a food he likes and has chosen. Letting a child dictate what he is given at every meal fails to guarantee that the food will be eaten and may result in an even more restricted diet, as he is likely to choose the same few foods over and over again.

You can allow him to make some choices in the supermarket, too, asking him, for example, which can of beans or which cucumber he thinks you ought to buy. At this age your toddler wants to make decisions for himself and you will need to develop the art of finding opportunities for him to exercise his independence, which will take some of the pressure off those times when you feel your decisions as a parent must be followed. Above all else, children want life to be 'fair' (although, admittedly, toddlers sometimes think this means having everything their own way). If you can point out to your child that he has been allowed to make some decisions for himself, you will feel stronger about insisting he does what you decide in other matters. And if your child sees that the principles of fair play are being upheld, he should be more amenable.

Sometimes the choices a child makes may be unconventional but not unhealthy. A child who wants, say, ham salad for breakfast is, in fact, choosing a healthy meal and one that would be normal in some other countries. How much you encourage or go along with such whims is up to you – but if he will eat what he has asked for, you may choose to admire his independence of mind.

Dawdling and vomiting

Dawdling over meals is common in this age group. Your child may spend time playing with his food, taking only tiny amounts at a time or putting it in his mouth and either not chewing it or seemingly chewing it forever. This can be infuriating if you want to get a meal finished and cleared away, but fascinating to the toddler who sees his mother helplessly trying to encourage him to eat. Unfortunately, making a fuss of his slowness is usually counterproductive – the toddler enjoys the fuss and becomes even slower to gain more attention and, for him, more diversions that distract him from eating.

Trying to force a child to eat may result in the whole lot being vomited back. Being sick is a talent that comes easily to children and is an unwise habit to allow to develop. Even if he is not sick, forcing food is likely to invite more trouble in the long run by making him dislike not only the specific food, but also mealtimes in general.

A better way of handling the situation is to allow him twenty minutes or so to eat. Then, if he will not respond after one or two suggestions that he eat a bit more, simply take his plate away. Be firm about making him wait until the next meal before he is allowed to eat again, otherwise his appetite will be dulled at that time. If, however, this procedure results in tantrums that you cannot endure, then allow your child to have something like a piece of bread or a suitable leftover from a previous meal. In this way you can show him that you will let him eat if he is hungry, but that you are making the rules about what is an acceptable snack. If he really is hungry, and not simply trying to wheedle a favourite snack out of you, then he will very likely eat what you offer.

Will eat with someone else but not with you

Although appetite problems are common at this age, many are made worse when they become a continual issue between parent and child. It can be particularly annoying to a parent to find a child eats well – and maybe eats foods he is thought to dislike – when away from home in the company of a childminder or babysitter. Before you judge yourself as an inadequate parent, remember that a toddler does not usually have the very close emotional ties to his caretaker that are needed to make battles so attractive to him. As adults we are not so different, for we tend to take out our moods on those closest to us while showing more reserve in the company of others. If your child is like this, then the less fuss you make, the sooner he will get bored with this behaviour.

Refuses to chew

The ability to chew has little to do with the presence of teeth, and more to do with the maturity of the jaw action. A child begins to be able to chew in a somewhat limited fashion from about seven or eight months, but the chewing process is not well developed until about eighteen to twenty-four months, when the bottom jaw is able to move not only up and down and from side to side but also in a circular motion. Until this age, therefore, it is not unusual for children to pass out lumps of unchewed and undigested food in their bowel movements. Provided your toddler seems well, there is no cause for concern and nothing need be done about it.

However, refusing to chew is a common behaviour problem that has much in common with dawdling. If your toddler is capable of chewing a piece of bread or a crust of toast – or a biscuit! – then he is obviously capable of chewing, but does not always choose to do so. Sometimes a toddler who won't chew is expressing a preference for the sorts of foods that are smooth and free of lumps. If he likes the taste of a particular brand of baby food or he has been used for too long to foods that have been finely blended in a liquidizer, then he is probably trying to engineer it so that he always gets this kind of food to eat rather than ordinary family food.

Trying to get your child suddenly to switch from spoonfuls of smooth pap to lumpy mixtures is likely to meet with his resistance. You can go along with his preference to some extent, but if he is eating a lot of manufactured foods, which tend to have a certain sameness about them, compromise by putting a portion of the family dish – particularly the meat part, which is often chewier, or unfamiliar vegetables – into a food blender. The resulting purée or sauce is a useful way of introducing your toddler to new foods and flavours while retaining the familiar texture.

If he is willing to eat foods that he can pick up with his fingers, you can give him pieces of cooked vegetable, pasta or rice, or chunks of apple, carrot or cucumber to nibble at the beginning of a meal when he is hungriest. Once he is eating these, you can put other foods that need to be chewed on his plate. If you are serving a sauce or a gravy, put it under the food so that the child can easily identify what is on his plate, as he is likely to be suspicious of 'disguised lumps'.

Miserable at meal times

A child who becomes withdrawn or starts to cry at the beginning of a meal makes it an occasion that has to be endured rather than enjoyed. The longer such a state of affairs continues, the harder it is to break the tension that the sight of food creates.

First you need to work out why meals are a source of friction. The most likely cause at this age is your concern that the child is eating very messily or has a poor appetite. Remember that most children are likely to be messy eaters until at least three. The mess can be accidental or deliberate; some children seem to need to get into their food a bit before they can get their food into them. See p. 41 for suggestions for keeping the mess within manageable limits. If poor appetite is the problem, see pp. 41–4.

A toddler who is feeling nagged at mealtimes is more likely to behave better when he can get a bit of peace. He is likely to respond best with the minimum of fuss – neither too much praise when he does eat nor any censure when he doesn't. You can also help by serving him a very small portion and leaving him to feed himself while you get on with something else near by, but preferably out of his sight. Give him a reasonable length of time – about fifteen or twenty minutes – then ask him if he has had enough (whether he has eaten anything or not) and let him get down. It may take a bit of time for him to unwind, so don't expect an immediate improvement. In the meantime give him opportunities to play with food away from the meal table so that he can get interested in it under less fraught circumstances. For example, you could give him small pieces of bread and salad vegetables for a doll's picnic and you can let him help you cook.

'Bad' table manners

Eating out or in the company of visitors is likely to be a trial for a toddler. He will not only be much more interested in all the new 'toys' (including other people and their ornaments) than the food, but he is also likely to become extremely frustrated if he cannot command his parents' full attention whenever he wants it. He may revel in the opportunity of having a larger audience to view his antics, and the more unused other people are to children, the greater the attention he is likely to attract.

It is unrealistic to expect very young children to eat tidily and quietly. If you have to take him with you when you go out to eat, give him his meal first, either before you go out or before everyone else eats. If you are in another person's home and your child can be fed out of sight of other adults, his eating won't give rise to comment and you will feel less obliged to keep trying to discipline him. If you are at a restaurant, where it may not be possible to let him eat separately, give him something, like a bread roll, that is easy to eat in his hands and involves no waiting. Bread is an excellent basis for a meal and you can later supplement it with items from your plate, thus avoiding the expense of a child-sized portion.

Of course, a child needs to learn to eat in company eventually, but at this age he may not be ready and, if you insist, you risk causing him to behave even more badly than he might otherwise.

Refuses to give up breast or bottle

Toddlers often have comfort rituals or objects, of which the breast or bottle may be one. The longer an infant sucks from the bottle or breast, the harder it is to break the habit. A baby who goes to sleep with a bottle may grow into a toddler who insists on keeping the bottle in bed with him or wandering around with a bottle always in his hand or mouth. And the baby who goes to sleep on the breast may find it difficult as a toddler to get back to sleep in the night unless he has a breast-feed. The older the child, the more help he is likely to need to give up the breast or the bottle.

There is no need to feel guilty about trying to wean your child from this comfort habit, but you can help him give it up or find an acceptable substitute only if you really want to. If you really enjoy breast- or bottle-feeding and you feel there is no harm being done, then why not continue to enjoy it until the time it either stops naturally or you decide it is becoming just a habit from which neither of you gets any special pleasure. Often, another pregnancy provides the motive for weaning a toddler.

If you do want to make the break, first work out when and why the breast or bottle is being used. Your toddler may be resorting to sucking when he is bored, unhappy, tired, needs to settle to sleep or simply because he enjoys a cuddle. Depending on how often your toddler sucks, it is probably better to tackle each of these problems separately.

A toddler who is bored should not be encouraged to suck simply to keep him quiet – he needs to be occupied with the stimulation of play, being read to and getting out and about. Use similar means to distract him if he wants the breast or bottle because he is momentarily upset about a fall or the loss of a toy. He will need to be able to rely on other means of comfort, such as cuddles and soothing words, when he goes to playgroup or nursery school.

Teasing him for still having the bottle or breast or making only half-hearted attempts to discourage him may fuel his determination to hang onto his love object. It will become more valuable to him if he thinks you are trying to take it away. If you have already been having a tug of war over the bottle or breast, give up nagging him about it for a couple of weeks, letting him have it whenever he asks. This will help him regain his trust and allow you a bit of time to plan how you are going to help him wean. In the meantime you could, for example, make a couple of times during the day when you sit and have a quiet cuddle with your child while watching a special television programme. When this routine has become established, you can then tell him that sucking is done only, say, after tea when he is tired or that it is a special kind of morning cuddle you have together.

Although babies can sometimes be weaned in a matter of weeks, it is likely to take much longer in the case of a toddler. When you are sure he is able – and merely unwilling – to do without the bottle or breast, you will have the confidence to be firm about your decision. You will probably have to expect tantrums for a few days, but if he sees that you really are determined and that he is not getting any less love or attention, he will feel secure, although possibly somewhat cross for a bit!

Chapter 6
From three to five years

From about three years of age a child is becoming increasingly independent. Because he can be relied on to look after his own needs in many ways, he can be independent of you for short periods, to go to playgroup or nursery school and to play at a friend's house. He is capable of understanding the meaning of rules much better and, although he may not always obey you, he enjoys familiar routines and customs, sometimes insisting that they are followed slavishly.

Patterns of development

At this age the things your toddler can do for himself – allowing for inevitable mishaps – include undressing and, later, dressing, going to the lavatory, washing his hands, helping with the washing-up, fetching items from the refrigerator, reminding you of things to put on the shopping list and laying the table. And what he is able to do, he is often insistent about doing. You may have to restrain yourself from interfering when he carries full milk bottles or wants to mix his own cakes, put washing powder in the machine, empty flour bags into the flour bin and roll out pastry. On the other hand, when there is a task you want him to do, such as tidy his toys, dress himself, use a knife and fork, drink from a cup rather than a beaker or even feed himself, he may act as if he is totally helpless, as taking the initiative is half the fun. Four-year-olds can be particularly self-willed, though by five children are usually a bit more sensible.

From about the age of three, your child's pot belly gradually disappears, his legs lengthen, and he becomes less clumsy and more active. His personality is emerging more clearly too, and you will find yourself and others gradually changing from saying 'He's at that age . . .' to 'He's that sort of child'. Every type of personality has its advantages and disadvantages. A lively, adventurous child may find it impossible to sit still or eat tidily but be willing to try new foods, whereas a quiet, shy child may have good table manners but be a fussy eater. This is not to say that all introverts are faddy eaters or that all extroverts have good appetites, but that a child's personality is bound to be expressed in some way in every facet of his life, including how and what he eats.

Between the ages of three and five a first-born child begins to discover the outside world (other children are usually made aware somewhat earlier). He soon learns that other people may eat different foods and have different sorts of drinks, and eat at different times. He will start to recognize places that sell hamburgers, vans that sell ice cream and shops that sell sweets. Even if he is not exposed to advertisements on television, he will begin to learn about delights that other children experience and expect to sample them himself.

Common eating problems

Likes and dislikes

Why do most young children seem to like certain foods, such as fish fingers, baked beans, jelly, chips, sausages, yoghurt and hamburgers, and commonly dislike others, including meat, eggs and vegetables – particularly green ones? The shapes, flavours and colours of these foods undoubtedly play a part in the choices children make, and so do their parents' attitudes.

The foods that most young children tend to dislike are the very ones that their parents think are particularly 'good' or healthy, while foods that are popular with children are usually the sort that parents feel less concerned about. For example, a parent will probably throw away a bit of uneaten bread or biscuit without a comment, but wave uneaten pieces of meat or vegetables on a spoon under a child's nose, saying either that meat is 'good' for him or that it is a shame to waste 'good' food. Thus a child may reject a food because of the pressure he is under to eat it rather than because of its taste.

Similarly, a child who is reluctant to try new foods at home or when out visiting may be more willing to experiment in a fast-food restaurant. In her own or someone else's home a parent may be anxious that her child will appreciate the food on offer, and may be even more anxious that he won't drop it on the hostess's clean floor or carpet. In a fast-food restaurant, on the other hand, there is no one to be offended if the food is not eaten and there are staff to clean up any mess. The child also has full permission to eat with his fingers. His parents not only take less notice of what he eats and nag less, but may also indicate that the food is a treat either by telling the child so or by commenting that they cannot understand why he should like such a disgusting drink or garish sauce! These relaxed circumstances are conducive to a child trying, and getting to like, unfamiliar tastes. Even a child who rejects a strong-tasting relish or an overly sweet drink at first may come to like it after a few more tries.

Poor appetite

Poor appetites are still common among three- and four-year-olds, although many children gradually grow out of this stage. You can help your child grow up by treating his poor appetite like any other phase in his development. He will develop a reasonable appetite naturally if you do not inhibit him by always refusing to let him decide what and how much he wants to eat.

By the time he is five, having seen him survive and thrive despite three or four years of poor eating, you will probably feel less worried about his appetite and more concerned about how he is coping with starting school. And being at school all day, and therefore unable to eat between meals, will help put an edge on his appetite.

Filling up on sweets and biscuits

By the time a child is four or five he is capable of getting food for himself. If he wants something to eat or drink, he knows how to help himself from the refrigerator, fruit bowl or bread bin, and by turning on a tap, unscrewing a bottle top or constructing 'ladders' to reach forbidden foods. You may find that, instead of refusing food, your child will take every opportunity to fill up on biscuits, crisps, sweets and ice cream. How many such opportunities he has will depend to some extent on whether he attends playgroup or school, and to some extent on the behaviour of the people he visits or who visit him.

A playgroup or nursery school may offer children a drink and a biscuit mid-morning or allow children to bring sweets to share on their birthday – and there can be a lot of birthdays to celebrate in one playgroup. If your child frequently comes home having had a snack, speak to the teacher or playgroup leader. Some playgroups will provide only milk to drink and make a rule – to the relief of many mothers – that children are not allowed to bring food to school, but can celebrate birthdays with a special song or activity. If your playgroup is not prepared to take this line, you can ask that your child be allowed only one sweet or crisp.

If you go to a mother and toddler group where biscuits and drinks are on offer, sound out the other mothers about stopping between-meal snacks. The chances are that a number of them will share your concern but have felt reluctant to take the initiative. If so, you will feel more confident about raising the matter for discussion. If the other parents are not willing to give up squash and mid-morning biscuits, they may be prepared to exchange them for a healthy snack, such as milk and a piece of fruit. Even if you don't succeed immediately, you will have drawn other people's attention to the existence of the problem, and they may feel differently when they have had time to think about your suggestion. In the meantime you could bring your own snack for your child, choosing the sort of food you would give him at mealtimes, such as a sandwich, breadsticks or a slice of bread cut into the shape of a gingerbread man.

Playgroup or nursery school is fairly neutral ground compared with visiting someone, particularly if it is someone you do not know well. When you take your child to visit other children, some form of refreshment is usually offered out of politeness, and it will probably be of the 'treat' variety – if only so that the mothers can enjoy it. On such occasions it can be difficult to restrict the number of biscuits or crisps your child eats.

If you are invited to another person's home for tea and you know it is likely that your child will be offered only cakes and biscuits, give him something like a sandwich or piece of cheese and an apple to eat before you go out. If he fills himself up before being tempted by sweet things, he may be satisfied with one biscuit rather than several. You will also have the satisfaction of knowing that he has eaten a meal that he otherwise might not have had room for.

Friends and relatives can cause problems if they bring sweets when they visit you, particularly if they try to persuade you that a few sweets 'once in a while' won't hurt. True, occasionally eating sweets and biscuits won't hurt, but by the time several people have offered them over the course of a few days, they no longer are 'once in a while'. The only way to prevent these temptations is to tackle them, tactfully, at the source.

Relatives can be very resistant to suggestions that they risk 'spoiling' your child, for spoiling is probably precisely what they want to do. It is important to realize that grandparents, aunts and uncles often want to enjoy a special relationship with your child. They like to know that he looks forward to their visits – even if it is only out of greed for what they bring with them! This perfectly natural wish on the part of relatives can be anticipated and channelled into an acceptable form of expression before the habit of bringing sweets is developed and needs to be broken. Think of a way in which each set of relatives can express the specialness of their relationship with your child. For example, one pair of grandparents might like to buy your child a special piggy bank and save pennies for him to put in it at each visit. Then every couple of months they can make a point of going out together to spend whatever has been saved on a special toy. The other grandparents might like to keep a 'magic' box or drawer in which a young child could find a small toy or book. An older child could be started on a special collection of things such as stamps, geological specimens, or model animals.

It is also worth explaining even to a young child why sweets and other sugary items are bad for his teeth. Your dentist will probably be delighted to reinforce this message. You may then be rewarded like one mother who overheard her son telling his granny that it was very naughty of her to give him sweets, as they might make his teeth sore. The granny was mortified and was heard begging forgiveness from her three-year-old grandson.

Convenience foods

Convenience foods tend to have a rather poor reputation for wholesomeness. This is a result of the huge increase in public awareness about nutrition and health and the subsequent warnings from health professionals and consumer organizations concerning the role of salt, sugar, saturated fats and artificial additives in the diet. If your child eats little but does enjoy such items as crisps, sausages, instant puddings and tomato ketchup, you may find yourself in a quandary: relieved that the child will eat, if only from a limited selection of foods, and concerned that such foods are not as good for him as others. Healthy eating is discussed in more detail in Chapter 8.

Although a healthy diet is obviously desirable, bear in mind that you can probably effectively tackle only one eating problem at a time. And a short period of less-than-perfect eating is unlikely to be any more harmful than a poor appetite. This is not to say that you should allow your child to dictate to you which foods he is prepared to eat – which would create problems rather than solve them – but you can afford to be more relaxed about some of the foods he eats until you are confident that he is healthy and able to eat a sufficient amount to keep him that way.

If convenience foods are to be regular items in your child's diet, take a positive attitude towards them.

Although by and large, convenience foods tend to be saltier, sweeter and have more artificial ingredients than home-prepared foods, they do vary considerably. An enormous number of products that claim, variously, to be low in fat, sugar or salt or free of artificial additives are now available. If your child will eat only commercially produced fish fingers, yoghurt and spaghetti shapes, you can at least choose varieties that have no artificial colourings and get their flavours from real food ingredients rather than flavouring extracts. Some convenience foods, such as fish fingers and baked beans, are wholesome and deserve much the same respect from the nutritional point of view as fresh foods. However, the very acceptability of some convenience foods should not stop you from encouraging your child to extend his tastes, as he will learn to try new foods only if he has regular access to a variety of them.

Lack of variety

A varied diet not only helps ensure sufficient quantities of essential nutrients, but also is a great social advantage, as other mothers may be reluctant to invite fussy eaters to share a meal with their children.

Giving your child as much opportunity to look after his own needs and suggesting – but not insisting – that he take just a taste of a new food, will encourage him to be more adventurous in his food habits. Offer him, for at least one meal in the day, the food that the rest of the family is eating. Invite him to serve himself, and if he does not want the meat or the vegetables, ask him to put a token amount on his plate even if he leaves it uneaten. Both you and he will get more satisfaction if he eats as much as he has taken, than if he takes a larger amount and seems to eat only a little of it. You may be so pleased to see a clean or nearly clean plate at the end of the meal that it may help you forget how little was on it to begin with. You may even feel inclined to give him an approving look rather than one of despair!

Serving extra potatoes, bread or another filling food that he finds acceptable will help him feel less threatened by a new food because he does not have to choose between eating it and going hungry; if there are no alternatives, the only choice open to a child is not to eat. He also needs to see you try new foods, which might, at the same time, help you understand how he feels.

Although eating a variety of foods at each meal is ideal, it is not essential. It is possible for small children to get a nutritionally balanced diet by eating a variety of foods over the course of a day, or even a week, and this is a more realistic goal. If your child eats toast at one meal, a banana at the next and a bowl of baked beans or an egg at another you can count this as a nutritionally varied diet which happens to have been taken over the course of a day.

Won't eat meat

Meat is not an essential component of the diet, but a child who refuses to eat meat can make life awkward for anyone who is not used to cooking nutritionally balanced vegetable-based meals. Simply dropping meat, or any major food group, from the diet without replacing it with its nutritional equivalent will result in an unbalanced, and therefore unhealthy, diet.

Since young children have only a limited understanding of what meat is, you might find some meat or fish product that your child will eat. A child who dislikes lumps of meat may like thinly sliced ham, fish fingers, mashed tuna fish or minced chicken. He may accept meat in the form of mince if it is well mixed with potato or rice, as in rissoles or risotto, or has been blended into a sauce for pasta.

If his powers of detecting meat are keen and he refuses even mince and meat sauce, you will need to prepare meatless meals that provide the complete proteins he needs. You can do this by serving pulses (beans, peas, lentils) with cereals (rice, corn, oats, pasta) or seeds and crushed nuts (including seed pastes, such as tahini, and peanut butter), or combining vegetables with cheese, eggs or milk. For example, you can serve rice with mixed bean and vegetable stew, cauliflower with cheese sauce, or pasta with lentil and tomato sauce, and milk puddings or yoghurt mixed with fruit to follow a first course of vegetables or sandwiches.

A child who doesn't eat meat is very unlikely to come to any harm, but you may feel stuck for ideas for his meals. There are many excellent vegetarian cookery books available, which will provide plenty of suggestions for alternatives to ring the changes.

Won't eat vegetables

The word vegetables refers to a wide range of foods, from substantial items such as potatoes and baked beans to light salad ingredients such as lettuce, and is even used to refer to some fruits, such as tomatoes. Vegetables are important in the diet because they contribute fibre and a variety of vitamins and minerals. Potatoes, and some other root vegetables, are also filling and make a useful contribution to the calorie content of a meal, while vegetables such as cabbage and cucumber, with an even higher water content, contribute relatively few calories.

Although potatoes, if eaten in sufficient quantity,

could satisfy virtually all of an adult's nutritional requirements, they are not as valuable in a child's diet
because of the small amounts a child can normally
consume. If a child dislikes potatoes, rice, pasta and
bread are alternatives.

If your toddler won't eat green vegetables, concentrate on red and yellow vegetables such as carrots, sweet
corn, tomato and sweet potato. He may prefer raw
vegetables he can hold in his hands, such as large
chunks of cucumber, carrot sticks, rings of red and
yellow peppers, cherry tomatoes, celery sticks,
cauliflower sprigs or raw peas. Salad vegetables may be
preferred because they taste sweet, but so do leeks,
swede, parsnips and coleslaw made with grated apple. If
you are going to introduce your child to a new range of
vegetables, try them one at a time in order not to
overwhelm him.

If he won't eat any whole vegetables, you may be able
to get some vegetables into his diet in the form of sauces
for pasta or by using finely blended vegetables as pizza
toppings. You can also substitute fruit for vegetables
and, failing that, give him fruit juice regularly or ask
your doctor about vitamin-mineral supplements.

In the meantime stop worrying and stop nagging him
about the fact he is not eating vegetables. Instead, keep
serving a selection of vegetables or salad items at mealtimes and leave him to help himself when he is ready. If
you put vegetables on his plate for him, he is likely to
continue feeling rebellious; if you don't provide any
vegetables, you take away the opportunity for him to
make a choice and you make vegetables seem even more
unfamiliar items to be suspicious of. Eventually, when
he thinks you have forgotten about vegetables or trusts
that you are not going to try to force him to eat them, he
is likely to serve himself some. He may not eat them

but, by putting them on his plate, he is finding them a bit more acceptable. If he does take a taste, he may spit it out either to see how you react or because it feels a bit strange and he wants to proceed cautiously.

Still being spoon-fed

Some four-year-old children are still being spoon-fed by their parents. Although children are usually fairly competent at feeding themselves with a spoon from the age of two, whether they choose to do so is another matter. Most children need to be helped from time to time – like scraping up the last couple of mouthfuls or at the times when they are hungry but overtired. But if you find yourself spoon-feeding your child at other times – and it will most likely be with foods he does not like – then he is simply enjoying you babying him. Some children are particularly fond of being cossetted from time to time and if spoon-feeding your four-year-old is your way of indulging this whim, then no lasting harm is likely to come from it. If, however, you are feeding him because you think he will not eat without your help, you can be sure that he is quite capable of feeding himself if he is hungry, although like most strong-willed four-year-olds he may protest vehemently and with plenty of tears in the hope that you will give in.

Bad table manners

Although teaching and maintaining good table manners is part of your general approach to managing your child's behaviour, it can be difficult to succeed if, at the same time, you are anxious because he does not eat enough. An intelligent child will often be only too happy to take advantage of your dilemma. You have to decide whether it is his poor eating or his bad behaviour that upsets you most. Many parents warn a child that if he does not sit still and eat reasonably tidily it is a signal that he has finished eating and he will not get any more food until the next meal. If you are anxious about a poor appetite, you will find it extremely difficult to carry out such a threat (which is essential if your child is to learn that you mean what you say). Instead, you could try sending your child into another room to eat or you could withdraw to eat elsewhere so that he is deprived both of an audience and your approval.

You can combine teaching courtesy at table with managing a poor appetite. A child likes to be allowed to perform adult activities and will thoroughly enjoy pouring out drinks from a jug, serving other people as well as himself, passing the marmalade or salad bowl and helping to clear the table. If he can also help prepare part of the meal – mixing the salad, cooking a pie or scrubbing the potatoes – he will be much more likely to be interested in the food and whether other people are enjoying it. His interest may not yet extend to eating much himself, but he should feel more positive about the process of eating, particularly if he receives a few compliments about his contribution. If this all seems like too much hard work – with all the inevitable spills and mishaps – remember that in a few years time you probably will be very thankful that your child can prepare a simple meal for himself.

Chapter 7
From five to ten years

Starting school signals the beginning of a new phase in your child's development, even if he has been to nursery school. He is entering a period when his thinking can change enormously and he is becoming increasingly independent in his thoughts and actions.

Patterns of development

You child's face is changing, thinning out and lengthening as the eyes, forehead and face gradually assume adult proportions. His baby teeth begin to fall out as his permanent teeth emerge, and differences in height between him and his classmates become more apparent. It is not unusual for a child to be skinny at this age and for his ribs to stick out, but as long as he continues to grow in height – and out of his clothes – from one year to the next, he is healthy.

Although not all children are natural athletes or graceful movers, they get a lot of pleasure from being active. They may get frustrated because they are not as good as they would like to be at a particular sport or activity, but they usually have tremendous reserves of determination and enthusiasm for practising a skill they feel is within their capabilities. They may also become discouraged if they are not allowed to jump and climb, if they are continually urged to acquire skills they are not ready for or if there is too much adult interference – particularly from a parent. Children enjoy opportunities to show off their physical skills and the feeling of freedom that their energetic, active play releases. But if they are made to feel incompetent or if the only form of exercise they take is obligatory, they may gradually cease to get any pleasure from it, and grow to dislike exercise to the detriment of their long-term health and well-being.

An active child will be developing the large muscles that help him to acquire new skills such as turning cartwheels and hopping, and improving the action of the small muscles such as those in the hand so that he is able to use a pencil and a knife and fork with much greater skill.

Peer group pressure

Probably the most startling change after your child turns five is his very strong need to identify with other children. He no longer wants the same toys as other children simply because they are fun, but because he finds it painful to feel different. As a parent you find yourself juggling with yet another set of conflicting demands. When he was a toddler you had to balance his need to be independent with your rules as his guardian. Now you have to balance his overwhelming desire to do what his friends and classmates do with your role in safeguarding his long-term interests. He is also now better able to think, to solve problems and to argue, and you may find yourself repeatedly being cornered by your own reasoning. He will probably demand to have the same food in his lunch-box or to stay up as late as someone else, arguing that other people's parents think it is all right.

Children of this age increasingly test rules to see whether they work and to see how you react. Now that he is more independent it is easier for him to break your rules, and you may find that your six-year-old has been watching a forbidden television programme on someone else's video or that he has been regularly accepting sweets from another child's lunch-box. As he gets older he will learn that rules are there for a reason and, although he may argue about them individually, he will develop the self-discipline to stick to them whether or not you are there to enforce them.

Hand in hand with this he will develop socially, moving from having a succession of continually changing friendships to being part of a smaller group and eventually to having just one or two close friends. In this way he will learn that people, in groups and individually, differ from each other. There will be limits to how different or individual he is prepared to be, as the desire – or peer-group pressure – to be like other children remains strong.

Encouraging skills with cutlery

Skills can develop only if a child is given the opportunity to practise them, and practice is no less important in learning to eat with a knife and fork than it is in learning to trace an intricate picture. Although a four-year-old should be able to handle a knife and fork, some children still have to have their food cut up for them by the time they start school. Although a certain amount of clumsiness is normal, it is also easy to discourage a child's development in this area if you always cut his food for him before he asks for help. If you are concerned that his whole plate might end up on the floor as he tries to cut his meat, then cut the awkward foods for him but get him to cut soft foods like potatoes and fish fingers so that he learns to use a knife. You can also encourage him to spread his own bread long before he gets on to tackling the intricacies of dissecting a chicken leg.

Food worries

On the whole, school-age children consider food important and the poor appetite of the early years will have developed into a healthy hunger and frequent requests to know when the next meal is coming. If you have a child who still eats little but is obviously healthy, you can probably now accept that a small appetite is normal for him. But worries about food are by no means over. Not only may the familiar problem of food fads still be present, but you may also face problems about school dinners, packed lunches and whether your child will eat the foods you think are good for him. As he gets older he may develop an earnest wish to become a vegetarian, and an overweight child may put himself on a diet in his desperation to become less of an object of mockery amongst his contemporaries.

School dinners and packed lunches

One of the first decisions to be made when your child starts school is whether he should eat school dinners, take packed lunches or go home for lunch. Your decision will depend to a large extent on the policy of the school, your own circumstances and, of course, what you think is in your child's best interests.

School dinners are not simply a matter of the kind of food available. They also mean eating in noisy surroundings with huge numbers of other children; being supervised by adults who may have very different rules about children and food than those set at home; sometimes being faced with unfamiliar or disliked foods; and lengthy sessions in the playground, with all the rough and tumble that this involves. Thus, eating at school can be a tremendously exciting and sometimes nerve-wracking adventure at first, and a major source of problems, which can become the focus of many of your child's worries about school.

If your child develops an anxiety about school meals, first ask the meal supervisors to check whether or not he usually does eat his food. If he is eating little and you think the reason is related to the quality of the meals, find out whether there is a district policy about what is on the menus. If there are guidelines, find out from your local health education unit the name of the community dietician attached to your health authority. Ask her whether she thinks the menus are satisfactory and, if not, whether she has any influence on them. A community dietician should be able to provide examples of good meals for your school caterers to consider. If there is general dissatisfaction among parents and children about school dinners, take up the matter with your Parent Teacher Association.

The school food may be good and popular with other children, and it may not be the food that is the real cause of your child's anxiety. Ask his teacher and whoever is in charge of the playground to keep an eye on him and let you know if he seems to have any problems. Your child may, in fact, be coping well at school, but just need some reassurance that he is doing all right. In such circumstances school dinners may be a convenient scapegoat for his worries, particularly if food is a subject he knows will guarantee your attention.

Packed lunches are not necessarily an easy alternative to school dinners. It is all very well providing a picnic once in a while, but finding ideas for sixty or more picnics a term takes some advance planning. A packed lunch should be the equivalent of a cold meal, not simply a fill-in snack before the child gets home from school. You need to think of at least five different kinds of cold meals – one for each day of the school week. Suitable foods are chicken drumsticks, cold sausages, squares of pâté, baked beans, sweet corn, chopped boiled potatoes, pasta or rice salads, wedges of quiche, vegetable salads, sandwiches, filled rolls or pitta bread, nuts and raisins, yoghurt, fruit cake and digestive or savoury biscuits and cheese.

Some of these foods – the chicken, fruit cake, bread rolls, sausages and even the quiche (provided it is defrosted carefully so that the pastry does not go soggy) – can be cooked in bulk in advance and frozen in individual portions. Ideally, they should be taken out of the freezer to defrost the night before they are needed, but small portions should be defrosted by midday if they are taken from the freezer early in the morning. Cans of beans and sweet corn are easily stored and if you also make a regular habit of buying salad vegetables, you should have plenty of materials from which to produce a packed lunch. It is also worth making a habit of cooking one or two extra potatoes each day as they can make a useful addition – particularly if the bread has run out!

At night prepare the next day's lunch in a shallow plastic box with a snap-on lid and put it in the refrigerator. Since the contents of the lunch-box are likely to get all mixed up in the course of being taken to school, it is best to include salad vegetables in mixed salads (for example, rice, mushroom, peanuts, celery, ham and peppers) or as finger foods (such as carrot, celery and cucumber sticks) and to wrap fragile items like pieces of savoury pie separately in foil or film. Put sloppy items such as baked beans or a salad with dressing in a small separate container with a snap-on lid, such as an old cottage cheese carton. Add a piece of fruit – an apple, pear, quartered orange, banana or melon wedge – or a tub of soft fruit and, for a hungry child, a yoghurt or some fruit cake or cheese and biscuits together with cutlery, a napkin and a drink if the school does not provide water.

Sandwiches – although excellent foods – can get monotonous, so use them for the days when you haven't been able to prepare a meal the night before. Suitable sandwich fillings include cottage cheese and pineapple, cheese, ham, peanut butter, tuna, egg, chicken, sardine, diced salad vegetables in low-fat mayonnaise or salad dressing and ricotta cheese, grated cheese and carrot, and low-fat pâtés. Bread does not always have to be turned into sandwiches and a roll or a hunk of bread is a good addition to any lunch-box.

It is easy to fall into the trap of asking your child what he wants. Letting him always direct what goes into his lunch-box is not a good idea: he may have a more limited repertoire of suggestions than you and he may try to persuade you to give him all sorts of 'fun' foods you would not normally provide for his meals. Some schools give dietary guidelines to parents that, for example, forbid the inclusion of sweets and chocolate biscuits. It should also be the responsibility of the staff supervising meals to check that each child eats a reasonable amount of what is in his packed lunch and to make sure that no child swaps the contents of his lunch-box with another child.

No breakfast

A good breakfast has long been advocated by many nutritionists, doctors and interested food manufacturers as an essential start to the day. Without it, parents have been warned, their children's concentration and work performance at school will suffer. A parent, who is naturally anxious that her child should do well at school, is instantly vulnerable to such threats. There is, however, little evidence to substantiate these claims. Briefly, breakfast seems to be important – as far as concentration and performance are concerned – only if it is eaten habitually. A person who *never* has breakfast is unlikely to suffer, as the body can adjust to many different patterns of eating. If your child has a very small appetite at the beginning of the day and it gradually improves as the day goes on so that by evening he eats a good-sized meal, it is unlikely that you have anything to worry about.

Obviously, however, breakfast is important to a child who is hungry early in the morning or who gets hungry well before the midday meal. A little hunger may sharpen the wits, but if your child misses breakfast because he gets up too late each day and he then gets hungry at school, it is common sense that his mind will be more on his stomach than on his school work.

An easy way to check your child's need for breakfast is to compare his breakfast-eating habits on school days and at weekends and in the holidays. If he eats breakfast on days when there is no school, then he probably does need to eat something at the beginning of the school day too. An earlier rising time (and an equally earlier bed-time) may help by giving him time both to play and get dressed in a reasonably unhurried manner. When he has been awake for about an hour, he is much more likely to feel hungry, and if he has been able to start the day in a reasonably relaxed, enjoyable way he will feel encouraged to eat. If he finds the usual breakfast foods boring, try offering him yoghurt and a banana, a sandwich, baked beans and a pancake, or a plain bread roll with a cup of hot chocolate or a milk shake.

It is also worth finding out whether there is anything troubling him at school, which is putting him off his breakfast. If not, he may simply not be a 'morning' person and is using a fuss about breakfast as a way of making the most of his grumpiness. In that case the less notice you take, the better. You could suggest that he gets his breakfast in peace on his own before everyone else wants to use the kitchen. Most children are sufficiently uninterested in clearing up after themselves for you to be able to see what he has had without needing to ask and so drawing attention to whether or not he has eaten.

Sweets

It is possible for a child to reach the age of two or so without having any idea what a sweet is. However, once he starts to meet other children, he soon learns that sweets are coveted treasures.

Sweets are loved for all sorts of reasons, not just their physical characteristics of shape, colour and taste. They are treats, rewards, bribes, objects to barter and symbols of friendship. Children share sweets or withhold them as a way of demonstrating who their friends are at the moment, and barter them in order to exchange pleasures and form new friendships: 'I'll let you have a piece of chocolate if you let me have a go with your car', and so on. Sweets also provide children with an opportunity to break certain adult rules. They may be shared in the most unhygienic circumstances: 'Two sucks of your gobstopper for two licks of my lolly'; and they are usually eaten between meals. Sweets are generally cheap enough to be bought with pocket money, and, in many ways, are a form of currency in childhood, which many adults, whether consciously or not, recognize and endorse to the annoyance of those parents who worry about their children's teeth or poor appetites.

Unfortunately, with all that sweets symbolize, warnings about the possible effects on teeth and health may fall on deaf ears or even enhance the attractions of the 'forbidden fruit'. Because sweets are not usually eaten simply to satisfy hunger, fruit or raw vegetables will not always be an acceptable substitute, with the possible exception of dried fruit, such as raisins. However, since dried fruits have a high sugar content, they offer little advantage over conventional sweets, at least in terms of dental health. But sweets are not the only form of childhood currency – there are stickers, badges, conkers, shells and toys. You can point out these alternatives to your child so that you do not feel guilty about seeming to be the only parent who deprives her child of sweets.

You can also explain to other children that sweets harm the teeth (but don't place too much emphasis on teeth falling out, as this may act as a positive incentive to the under-eights!) and point out that your child is not an object of pity, as on the few occasions when he does get sweets, they seem even more of a treat. You may have to put up with the reputation of being a mother who doesn't allow sweets, but there may be other parents who will be grateful that you are prepared to take a lead that they can follow.

If you find that, despite your efforts, your child still seems to be getting regular supplies of sweets, it is probably wisest to permit them but, wherever possible, within certain limitations. For example, keep any sweets he has acquired until one time in the day when he may eat them, which is less harmful to his teeth than sucking them at intervals throughout the day.

Sweets provide a useful opportunity to encourage a

child to discuss a matter about which you and he may not see eye to eye. If you show that you have listened to him and that you do understand his feelings, you may be able to reach a compromise. For example, you might suggest to an eight-year-old that while you choose not to give him and his friends sweets, he is now old enough to spend a small proportion of his pocket money on sweets if he wishes to do so.

Deciding to be a vegetarian

A child who wants to be a vegetarian is likely to be a 'problem' only if you and the rest of your family are fond of meat and/or have little familiarity with vegetarian dishes. Even if you do not consider yourself a meat-eater, your food habits may be very strongly affected by the traditional role of meat in the diet.

In Western industrialized countries, the diet is traditionally meat-oriented. Most of us have been taught, consciously or subconsciously, to decide what the meat part of the meal will be and let that dictate which vegetables will accompany it. For this reason, if no other, having a vegetarian in the family can seem disturbing, an upset out of all proportion to the relative nutritional importance of meat.

A child's natural love of animals often leads to a wider interest in their welfare. Therefore it is, perhaps, not surprising if a child who loves a pet as much as any other member of the family begins to think it cruel to kill animals for food. If your child feels like this, he is likely to have very strong feelings on the subject, which you will not be able to treat lightly. However, a child may have his own interpretation of what being vegetarian means, and may find certain animal foods acceptable. Thus he may reject a joint of meat, and pieces of meat with names such as rabbit, duck, chicken or lamb, but accept hamburgers and sausages because they don't look or sound like animals that were once alive.

If you enjoy meat, you might be tempted to try to repress your child's inclination to become a vegetarian. However, if he is determined not to eat meat, you cannot expect him to live on a diet of vegetables with a chunk of cheese or an egg at every meal in the hope that he will soon grow bored of such a monotonous diet. Since children tend to be conservative eaters, you can be quite certain that you will get bored of serving him the same old foods long before he gets tired of eating them.

Vegetarianism is no longer considered odd and it is not unhealthy, so you may find it easier to let your child try a vegetarian diet than to fight it. If so, the problem you face is how to provide meals that meet his needs as a vegetarian without requiring the rest of the family to give up meat if they don't want to. In fact, a vegetarian in the family, rather than restricting the family's choice of food, can give an often much-needed stimulus to expanding your culinary repertoire.

A vegetarian diet involves a different way of structuring a meal than one based on meat. In a traditional meat-based cuisine meat is the focal point of the meal and vegetables are merely an accompaniment. There are some vegetarians who cannot get away from this meal stereotype and as a result omelettes, cheese salads and nut cutlets – where eggs, cheese or nuts replace meat as the focal point of the meal – have become clichéd alternatives. This approach to vegetarianism results in a somewhat limited diet, and you will probably soon run out of ideas for meat substitutes. However, there are many excellent vegetarian cookery books available to help you create interesting and varied meals. They often include recipes for dishes from foreign cuisines in which meat, if eaten, plays only a subsidiary role. For example, in such traditional Italian dishes as pizza, risotto and spaghetti, the central part of the dish is bread, rice or pasta. This staple is then made interesting with vegetables, sauces, garlic and herbs – and occasionally a little meat. In the Chinese and Indian cuisines rice is the staple, and is usually accompanied by several other dishes served separately. In India and the Middle East pulses – that is, peas, beans and lentils – also play a major role in the diet. They are excellent sources of protein and dietary fibre, and are usually low in fat.

Instead of trying to adapt a meat-based meal for a vegetarian, you may find it easier to prepare a vegetarian meal and adapt it for those who like meat. For example, you can serve a hot savoury rice dish – made with onions, peppers, mushrooms, peas and nuts – and a salad, with a bowl of chopped ham, bacon or prawns for those who want meat; or prepare a vegetable stew, divide it into two serving dishes and add cubes of meat to one. You can also offer salads in which all the ingredients are served separately so that everyone can choose what he wants, rather than pick out the bits he doesn't like. Your other children may welcome more pizzas, vegetable-stuffed pancakes and baked potatoes without even noticing that they don't contain meat.

Foods that are useful standbys in the store cupboard for snacks and quick meals are baked beans, peas, sweet corn, peanut butter, nuts and raisins, as well as canned chick peas and lentils, which can be puréed with herbs and spices to make a spread or be used as a filling for a flan. You can also buy, or find recipes for, vegetarian pâtés and nut butters to use as sandwich fillings.

Whether or not you agree with your child's preferences, it is worth setting a time limit for the experiment. You can suggest that he tries a vegetarian diet for a month to see how he likes it. This not only shows him that you support him, but also gives him a date by which he can change his mind, if he wants to, without losing face. Depending on his reasons for becoming a vegetarian, he may then be prepared to accept the return of certain meat dishes.

Chapter 8
Healthy eating

Like all parents, you want your child to be healthy, and you worry if he does not eat much of anything, let alone a varied diet. Your worries and doubts can be fuelled by the emphasis on healthy eating in the mass media; by using tables of average heights and weights to evaluate your child's growth; and by comparing your child to others of the same age.

In the mass media reports on healthy eating the advice of doctors and nutritional experts to eat more of this and less of that is, of course, usually given in generalized terms. Therefore, it is not appropriate in every detail to every individual. For example, if you normally use very little salt on your food and eat a substantial amount of a variety of fresh fruit and vegetables, the advice to eat less salt and more fresh produce obviously does not apply to you. In the same way you may find that although articles on healthy eating advise giving toddlers low-fat products, such as semi-skimmed milk, your health visitor or doctor may tell you that *your* child still needs full-fat milk to ensure he gets enough calories. Thus you can see that it is important to know how the guidelines for healthy eating apply not only in general, but also specifically to your child.

Similarly, if you see a table of heights and weights that is based on averages, you have to remember that an average is simply the middle of a range. For example, the *average* two-year-old girl is supposed to be 85.6 cm (2 ft 9¼ in) tall and weigh 12.2 kg (26 lb 13 oz), but the *range* of heights considered normal for a girl this age is 79.4 cm to 91.8 cm (2 ft 7 in to 3 ft), and the range of normal weights is 9.7 kg to 14.9 kg (21 lb 5 oz to 32 lb 13 oz). Just as important in assessing your child's growth is how he looks and behaves. A healthy child is bright-eyed and active, with a lively interest and curiosity in things around him.

Comparing your child's eating habits with those of other children can also be misleading. Just as children vary in their growth rates, so they can vary in their nutritional needs. Research has shown, for example, that babies of the same size can vary threefold in the amount of milk they drink.[1] This means some babies need less milk than others to achieve the same growth, so you do not have to worry just because your baby drinks less than others you know.

Eating a healthful diet from birth is, of course, the ideal. Unhealthy eating habits increase the risk of health problems in later life, and the longer habits persist, the harder they are to change. But what is a healthy diet for a child? The medical evidence is not always clear-cut or conclusive. Some experts say, for example, that because coronary heart disease can be identified in childhood, prevention needs to start as soon as possible, while others argue that it may be foolish to try to reduce the amount of fats and sugars in the diet when a child is growing and at an age when food fads and poor appetites are common. Similarly, parents will probably see no problems, and considerable advantages, in teaching a child with a good appetite healthy eating habits from the beginning, while others may be more concerned that a child with a poor or faddy

[1] R. G. Whitehead, 'Principles involved in assessing energy, protein and micronutrient needs during infancy', *Proceedings of the Nutrition Society*, vol. 45, Sept. 1986, pp. 361–7.

appetite is eating enough even if the diet is not an ideal one. What experts do agree on are the basic nutritional requirements for a child.

Calories

Food and drink are the basic fuel from which the body extracts nutrients and energy, which it needs to grow, maintain itself and function. The amount of fuel, measured in calories, that people need varies considerably, depending on age, size, sex, amount of physical activity and metabolism. Some people have a metabolism that is highly efficient at storing, or 'saving' energy and need fewer calories than those whose bodies seem to use up or 'waste' a lot of energy. Whether one is born a 'saver' or a 'waster', the body's metabolism can change in certain circumstances. For example, during pregnancy the metabolism becomes more efficient at storing, or 'saving', so a pregnant woman does not necessarily have to eat more than she did before she conceived in order to provide the growing foetus with the energy and nutrients it needs.

It is of little consequence to the body what foods provide its calories. It can get them from proteins, fats and carbohydrates – starches and sugars – with almost equal ease. Fats are the most concentrated source of calories, providing twice as many calories weight for weight as proteins or carbohydrates. Fats and sugar are highly palatable and, used in moderation, can make the bulkier, plainer foods such as cereals and potatoes more interesting. However, if foods rich in fats and sugars are consumed in large quantities, they may replace other, more nutritious foods that provide the proteins, vitamins and minerals that the body also needs.

For example, a child who likes chocolate biscuits will,

if given the choice, be more likely to fill himself up on such a delicacy than eat a well-balanced meal. He will be satisfying his body's basic energy requirement, but not providing it with the other nutrients it needs.

Can a child choose?

Will a child, if left to himself, choose a healthy diet? Common sense suggests that if a child were offered a bag of sweets or a steak, he would most probably choose the sweets, because of their taste as well as their easiness to suck and hold. However, in the past some child-care manuals have suggested that children will eat what they need if left to themselves. This claim owes its origin to research in infants' eating habits carried out in America in the 1920s.[2]

The researcher – a paediatrician – studied the weaning progress of fifteen babies from between the ages of seven and ten months until they were two years old in what may be described as institutional care. At each meal the babies were given a tray containing between eleven and fourteen foods. The foods offered were raw and cooked meats; fish; unsweetened raw and cooked porridges made from various cereals; rye crispbread; bone marrow; raw and cooked eggs; fresh and soured whole milk; raw fruits and cooked apple; sea salt; and water. There were no processed foods, no sugar and no foods cooked with salt, and the infants were not allowed anything except water between meals. Each infant was fed in isolation except for the presence of a nurse, who showed no emotion, did not talk to the child and fed it

[2] Clara M. Davis, 'Self-selection of diets by newly weaned infants. An experimental study', *American Journal of Diseases of Children*, vol. 36, 1928, pp. 651–79.

only what it wanted. Not only were the children reported as thriving on this regime, but there were apparently no problems of poor appetite. Indeed, the researcher reported that the babies approached each meal with enthusiasm and produced little mess.

Clearly, these babies were brought up in a totally artificial environment, and although the result of the experiment is interesting, it does not have much relevance to children's normal eating habits. Children in a normal family situation are not isolated, they have an emotional relationship with the adults that look after them, and they are exposed to a vast range of processed, sweetened and highly flavoured foods and drinks on supermarket shelves, through advertising and through social contact with other children.

Probably the only conclusion that can be drawn from the American study is that a baby is capable of selecting a healthy diet for himself if he is offered only healthful foods and his parents, confident that they approve of the diet, are able to relax and let him make his choices.

Proteins

Although the human body can produce all the energy it needs from the proteins, fats and carbohydrates found in food, it can make the proteins it needs only from other protein. Every cell in the body contains some protein. The body needs continuous supplies of proteins to make new cells for body growth and to replace the cells that are worn away each day. Because children are growing rapidly they need proportionately more protein than adults. A newborn baby requires five times as much protein as an adult for every 450 grammes (1 lb) in weight. The body's protein requirement gradually decreases from the age of three months until after puberty, when it reaches the adult level.

Foods such as bread and cereal are good sources of proteins, but should not be swamped with fats or sugars. Many of the so-called high-protein foods – meat, milk, cheese and eggs – are frequently accompanied by a lot of fat. In the context of the diet as a whole they are not usually such important sources of proteins as they are often thought to be. For example, in a ham sandwich more protein is supplied by the bread than the ham.

Although a child needs relatively more protein than an adult, no special effort needs to be made to give it to him. The majority of people in Britain – children and adults – eat far more protein than they need; the surplus is converted into energy or stored as body fat. A child who satisfies his appetite by eating nutritious foods will get a sufficient quantity of protein. If, however, he were allowed to live exclusively on a diet of sweets and soft drinks, he would become deficient not only in proteins, but also in most of the vitamins and minerals as well.

Fats

As a highly concentrated source of calories, fats can be beneficial in the diet of a child who has a small appetite because they can boost the energy content of food without increasing the size of the portions. For example, a small knob of butter or margarine on a portion of carrots can increase the calorie content of the serving about threefold. Conversely, fats can add surplus calories to the diet of a child who is overweight.

Certain fats – known as the essential fatty acids – are necessary for the structure of the cells. However, the amount needed is so small that the danger of a deficiency is remote, as it is highly unlikely that anyone would find a diet devoid of fat palatable.

Diets rich in fat have increasingly been linked with coronary heart disease. Fats can be divided into saturates, monounsaturates and polyunsaturates. Cholesterol, which is a type of fat found naturally in the body as well as in some foods, becomes part of the plaque that accumulates in the arteries, causing them to narrow and harden. Saturated fats in the diet tend to increase the amount of cholesterol in the blood, while polyunsaturated fats (which contain the essential fatty acids) tend to reduce it – but at about half the rate that saturates increase it. Some scientists have argued that extra quantities of essential fatty acids will protect the body against heart disease, but this theory has not been generally accepted by medical experts.

Although heart disease may seem to be a problem of the middle-aged and elderly, it develops slowly over many years and the initial stages have been found in the arteries of children. British government medical experts advise that everyone over the age of five years should eat less of all fats, and particularly less saturated fats. That means not merely substituting polyunsaturated margarines and oils for saturated fats such as butter and lard, but reducing the amount of fried foods and high-fat dairy products you eat in favour of low-fat foods such as cereals, bread, beans, potatoes, fruit and vegetables.

Not all experts are agreed on whether children under five need or should have a low-fat diet. Babies start life on a high-fat diet, as half the calories in breast and formula milk are derived from fats, and as a general recommendation paediatricians advise that children under two years old should not be given semi-skimmed milk and should not be given fully skimmed milk under five years of age. Fat is still an important source of calories in the diet of toddlers and pre-school children, who must derive their full calorie needs from relatively small amounts of food.

If your child is growing and full of energy, you can be confident he is getting all the calories he needs. If he has a small appetite and you have been giving him a low-fat diet, you could try boosting his calorie intake by adding knobs of margarine to vegetables, spreading his bread with margarine and honey, and giving him whole milk to drink. If he does not seem any better or eats less because he is filled up more quickly by the richer food, it is unlikely that he was getting too few calories initially.

Carbohydrates

Starches, sugars and fibres are part of the spectrum of chemically related substances called carbohydrates, which the body uses to manufacture energy. Although carbohydrates share many chemical similarities, their role in the diet can be very different. Foods that are rich in starch, for example, such as potatoes, flour, oats and beans, are also good sources of vitamins and minerals. And since potatoes, flour and beans are also roughly three-quarters water, they are bulky, filling foods. In contrast, sugars supply no substantial nutrients, just calories. Sucrose, the kind of sugar found in the sugar bowl, is used in the preparation of sweets and sweetened foods and drinks. These foods are not particularly filling and their taste makes them easy to eat and 'more-ish' even if one is not hungry.

The human body does not need sucrose; it can manufacture energy just as well from starches and from the sugar in fruits and vegetables, which have the advantage of also providing vitamins, minerals, fibre and water. Although there is no evidence that a diet high in sugar is necessarily deficient in nutrients, it is common sense not to allow sugary foods and drinks to take the place of nourishing foods, particularly in the case of a child with a small appetite.

Sugar and teeth

Sugar is bad for teeth. Bacteria in the mouth feed on the sugar deposited on the teeth and produce an acid that destroys the enamel, and the new enamel on children's teeth is particularly vulnerable. Saliva is nature's mouthwash, but it takes time for the saliva to neutralize the acid. The more often sugar is in the mouth, the more difficult it is for the saliva to effectively neutralize it. It is, therefore, the frequency of sugar consumption and the length of time it remains in the mouth, rather than the quantity, that is harmful to teeth.

Although no one knows the precise number of onslaughts of sugar the mouth can cope with, most dentists would advise that sugary foods and drinks be restricted to mealtimes, when the saliva flow is increased and the other foods help to remove sugar from the mouth. Fresh and dried fruit and fruit juice are just as bad for teeth as sweets and biscuits, and should be avoided between meals. Because saliva flow is reduced at night it is important that children do not have sweet drinks just before going to bed or during the night.

Foods containing protein seem to have a protective effect, which is why milk, despite containing the sugar lactose, does not seem to harm the teeth. Although in theory a child ought not to be at risk of harming his teeth if he eats a sugary biscuit followed by a drink of milk, dentists do not yet know whether this is so in practice. In the meantime you can help your child to have healthy teeth by brushing them twice a day with a fluoride toothpaste. Your dentist may suggest painting fluoride on the surfaces of the back teeth and advise you on the use of fluoride drops.

Fibre

Fibre is a collective name for a number of highly complex carbohydrates found only in plants and foods made from them. Different kinds of plant contain different fibres: the fibre in wholegrain cereals and flours, for example, is different from that in peas and beans or fruit and vegetables. The fibre in wholemeal bread and wholegrain cereals is particularly good at helping the intestines work properly. A baby who is fed only on milk does not need fibre, but introducing high-fibre foods, such as wholemeal bread, brown rice and wholemeal pasta, rather than the refined, 'white' equivalents, during weaning will start him on a healthful diet.

Although wholegrain foods are suitable for a baby, bran-enriched products are not, mainly because they tend to be filling without providing sufficient calories for a baby or a young child with a small appetite. There is no benefit to health in giving a baby bran-fortified products even as a remedy for constipation. Constipation, which is common when a baby starts solids, can be treated by feeding him fruit, particularly prunes and prune juice, and, in the case of an older baby or child, wholemeal bread.

Vitamins and minerals

All foods that provide protein also provide some vitamins and minerals, and fruits and vegetables are other good sources. The table on pp. 99–102 lists the principal vitamins and minerals needed by the body, some of the foods in which they are found and the amount a child needs each day. There is some evidence to suggest that children given a little more than the recommended amount of vitamin A – the equivalent of half a carrot a day – suffer fewer infections than other children.[3]

If your child eats very little or has a very faddy diet, ask your doctor if vitamin and mineral supplements are necessary. If the doctor recommends supplements, be sure to keep them, like other medicines, where a child cannot reach them, as vitamins A and D are highly poisonous in large doses.

Iron is the one mineral that is sometimes in short supply in a young child's diet, particularly at the stage of being weaned off fortified babyfoods onto the normal family diet. However, an iron intake that is low relative to the amounts recommended does not mean that a child will have an iron deficiency – that is, be anaemic. It is likely that other factors – such as anaemia in the mother during pregnancy and breast-feeding, and a prolonged milk-only diet followed by being weaned onto a mainly starchy diet – are important in producing anaemia in a child. A combination of all these factors is much less common in industrialized countries like Britain, where toddlers do not suffer from anaemia, than in parts of the developing world, where they do.

Salt

A baby's immature kidneys can cope with only a limited amount of sodium. Most of the sodium in food comes from salt that is added during or after preparation. Because too much sodium in a baby's diet can cause

[3] *Australian Paediatric Journal*, vol. 22, 1986, pp. 95–9.

dehydration, paediatricians advise against adding salt to a baby's food. For this reason many manufacturers do not add any salt to baby food products, and those that do follow internationally agreed guidelines so that the amounts added are tiny and within a safe limit.

The amount of salt in the diet is important after babyhood too, for research has shown that some adults may develop high blood pressure as a result of a high-salt diet. Unfortunately, there is no way of predicting which people, other than those who are overweight or have a family history of high blood pressure, are likely to develop this condition, and by the time it can be diagnosed, it will often have done considerable irreparable harm to the arteries. Studies have shown that most people eat larger quantities of salt than they need, and nutritionists now recommend that everyone reduces the amount of salt in their diet.

Since a baby is weaned onto a low-salt diet, you can continue his healthy eating habits as he is introduced to regular family meals by using less salt in cooking and at the table, and by avoiding giving him salty snack foods. If the rest of the family are used to salty foods, you will need to modify the use of salt gradually to give their taste-buds time to adjust. Using a salt grinder instead of a salt shaker on the table often helps to reduce salt consumption initially, as the same number of wrist actions produces less salt.

Additives

Despite extensive testing procedures, safety standards and numerous regulations and codes of practice, many people are concerned about the presence of additives in foods. They want to know, firstly, whether additives are absolutely safe and, secondly, whether the products that contain them are nutritionally inferior to those that do not.

Manufacturers point out that elaborate safety precautions exist to ensure that no food additive is any more harmful – and, indeed, probably less so – than the toxic substances that are present or can occur naturally in virtually all foods. Some additives are used to protect food against contaminants that might make it unsafe.

They also argue that many of the foods we buy would not be available without the use of additives. For example, without anti-caking agents, lubricants and anti-foaming agents, factory equipment would quickly get gummed up or blocked by food ingredients as they are mixed together. Unlike the domestic cook, food factories cannot stop their equipment to remedy these problems and still maintain the vast supplies of bread, baked beans, wrapped cheeses and other prepared foods the public has come to expect. Similarly, without anti-oxidants, humectants and other preservatives many foods would have a much shorter shelf-life, which means people would have to shop more often, there would be a higher level of waste by spoilage and so food would become more expensive.

Although all these points are fair, there are also products, including savoury snacks, sweets and instant desserts, that have more additives than recognizable foods in the list of ingredients, and some in which additives are used to dress up poor quality food.

Parents may also be concerned because some children have been shown to be sensitive to a number of additives (see Chapter 9), but practically all these children were also allergic to several common foods such as eggs, milk and wheat. In other words, a child is no more or less likely to be allergic to additives than to any other food.

The major vitamins and minerals: recommended daily amount (RDA)

Vitamins	Main function	Good food source	RDA (ages 1–11 yrs)*
Vitamin A – retinol (Carotene in plants is converted into A in the body)	Needed for growth of new cells – particularly those of skin, lungs, eyes and intestines	Carrots, vegetables such as spinach and broccoli, apricots, melon, liver, fish oils, kidney, milk, butter, cheese, eggs, margarine and baby foods.	450–575 micrograms
B vitamins B_1 – thiamin		Bread, particularly wholemeal, yeast extract, peas, beans, nuts, pork, oats, milk, potatoes, other vegetables and fruit.	½–1 milligramme
B_2 – riboflavin	Needed for the chemical release of energy from carbohydrate and protein	Liver, kidney, yoghurt, cheese, yeast extract, eggs, meat, mushrooms, bread (particularly wholemeal), fortified breakfast cereals.	½–1.2 milligrammes
Niacin		Liver, kidney, meat, fish, yeast extract, peanuts, peas, beans, bread (particularly wholemeal), vegetables, milk, fortified breakfast cereals.	5–14 milligrammes

The major vitamins and minerals (cont.)

Vitamins	Main function	Good food source	RDA (ages 1–11 yrs)*
B$_6$	Needed to help build rapidly dividing cells, like blood and nerve cells, and for building proteins.	Most animal and plant foods.	no RDA
B$_{12}$		Liver, kidney, sardines, meat, eggs, cheese, milk.	no RDA
Folate (Folic acid)		Fresh fruit like oranges and bananas, salad vegetables, other green vegetables, liver, kidney, beetroot, peanuts, wholemeal bread, eggs, some fish, fruit juice.	100–200 micrograms
Vitamin C – ascorbic acid	Maintain strength and elasticity of skin and connective tissue between the joints. Aids absorption of iron from food.	Fresh fruit and raw vegetables; in particular blackcurrants, green peppers, oranges, lemons, cauliflower, broccoli, sprouts, cabbage, new potatoes, fruit juice.	20–25 milligrammes
Vitamin D	Needed to lay down calcium in bones and for efficient action of heart muscle and nerves	Most important source is sunlight as very few foods contain D except fish liver oils and fortified baby foods. Tuna, salmon, sardines, eggs, liver and margarine provide a little.	10 microgrammes unless adequate exposure to sunlight.

Vitamins/ minerals	Main function	Good food source	RDA (ages 1–11 yrs)*
Vitamin E	Helps maintain the strength of cell membranes	Vegetable oils, margarines, eggs, butter, wholegrain cereals, broccoli.	no RDA
Vitamin K	Needed for normal clotting of the blood.	Produced by the action of bacteria in the intestines and also found in vegetables.	no RDA
Minerals			
Calcium	Most is laid down in the skeleton to give bones their strength and hardness. A small but vital amount is also needed for stimulating the action of muscles and nerves and for clotting of blood.	Milk, yoghurt, cheese, canned fish (if bones are eaten), hard water, green vegetables, peanuts, bread and flour.	600–700 milligrammes
Fluoride	Needed for strength of bones and tooth enamel	Found in only a few foods: seafood, soy beans, tea and in varying amounts in water.	no RDA

The major vitamins and minerals (cont.)

Vitamins	Main function	Good food source	RDA (ages 1–11 yrs)*
Iron	Present in blood; carries oxygen round the body.	The iron in food varies in its ability to be absorbed. Liver, meat and fish are the best sources. Vitamin C will help the absorption of iron from plant foods.	7–12 milligrammes

Zinc, iodine, sodium, potassium, phosphorus, chloride and magnesium are also needed but in relatively small amounts. They are found in the same foods as other minerals and vitamins.

* Figures from DHSS, *Recommended Daily Amounts of Food Energy and Nutrients for Groups of People in the UK*, London, HMSO, 1979.

The concern about the possible allergic effects of additives may be a manifestation of many parents' misgivings about the quality of some of the foods aimed at the children's market, where artificial colours and flavours are used to entice children to buy snack foods and drinks of very doubtful nutritional benefit. Even in the case of supposedly nourishing foods, such as yoghurts and certain drinks rich in vitamin C, the colour – judging from the stains around mouths and on clothes – sometimes appears far stronger in the products intended for children than in the 'adult' versions.

An increasing number of products are now being made without added colouring, preservatives or artificial flavours. This does not always mean that a product is free of all additives; thus a yoghurt that contains no added colouring may still contain a preservative. You can find out what a product does contain by reading the list of ingredients on the label.

Organically grown foods

Many people buy 'organically grown' foods in the belief that they are healthier and better tasting than the same items grown intensively, that is, with the aid of chemical fertilizers and pesticides. Since taste is a matter of individual preference, there is little to be gained from discussing it; suffice it to say that in taste tests people usually have not been able to tell the difference between organically and intensively grown produce. In addition, in Britain there is no legally enforceable definition of 'organically grown' food yet, so there is no guarantee that food thus labelled has been treated any differently from intensively grown food. It has to be taken on trust by the retailer and the consumer.

There are also no approved standards of quality for organically grown foods. You can visibly check the quality of fresh fruit and vegetables and not buy apples that are blemished or carrots that have holes, but this is not possible with pulses, dried fruit and grains. When sold loose, these goods not only are much more vulnerable to infestation and contamination from foreign objects and from bacteria and moulds that are invisible to the naked eye, but also may have no label or sign indicating where they were grown. If produce has been imported from a poor tropical country where it has been stored in hot, humid conditions, it could have become contaminated with mould by-products such as aflatoxins, which are highly poisonous. If you want to buy organically grown pulses, nuts or grains, it is best to choose packaged goods supplied by a well-known reputable producer or retailer. Such large companies are able to provide adequate storage and transport facilities even in tropical locations and will have a system of quality control.

Processed foods

Processed foods are not the recent phenomenon they are
sometimes thought to be. People have been making
fundamental alterations to their food since they discovered fire – and maybe even before. Some ancient
processing techniques, such as making bread from
ground wheat grains and cooking meat, not only improve the taste of the basic ingredients, but also make
them more digestible. Some more modern processes can
extract specific elements from one food so that they can
be used in or with others. Thus sugar extracted from
sugar beet, butter fat from cream and oil from soya beans
can be added to other foods to modify their taste and
texture. Today processing technology is so sophisticated it can break down raw materials to as near their
basic nutritional components as desired and rebuild
them in an endless variety of combinations.

Two foods that demonstrate the advantages such
technology can bring are baby milk formula and soft
margarine. Nowadays bottle-fed babies can thrive on a
formula that is far superior to ordinary cow's milk, and
babies with an allergy to cow's milk protein can be fed a
formula based on a protein extracted from soya beans.
The margarine industry has produced a soft spread made
from oil as an alternative to butter, which is processed
from liquid cream. Soft margarine has an easily manipu-
lated fat content, so that 'healthier' versions are possible, and it can be spread thinner more easily than hard
fats, which is an advantage for people who are trying to
keep their calorie intake down.

Unfortunately, the same technology can also be used
to process water, sugar, fats, cornstarch, colourings and
flavourings – and even air – to produce sweets, snacks
and meal 'extras', described by marketing people as 'fun'

foods, which provide relatively little of the nutrition found in the basic whole ingredients. In the context of a healthful diet of a variety of basic foods a few coloured and salted 'cornstarch puffs' or the occasional sticky confection of sugar and fat are unlikely to be of much consequence. However, when these items are consumed in such quantity that they replace basic foods in the diet, they are a cause for concern. For example, the average person in Britain gets nearly 40 per cent of the calories in his diet from fat, 20 per cent from sugar and 5 per cent from alcohol, which leaves the remaining 40 per cent to provide all the other necessary nutrients: vitamins, minerals, proteins and fibre.

Putting principles into practice

Your child will have a healthful diet if he eats enough wholesome food to satisfy his hunger. Even if has only a small appetite, he will almost certainly get all the nutrients he needs by eating some foods from each of the following food groups every day: cereals and grains, such as bread, rice and pasta; fresh fruit and vegetables; moderate quantities of milk, cheese and yoghurt; lean meat, poultry, fish and eggs; pulses, nuts and seeds; and only small amounts of sugar and fats, such as butter, oil and margarine. In addition, plenty of exercise and fresh air will encourage a healthy appetite, maintain fitness and ensure adequate supplies of Vitamin D from the action of sunlight on the skin.

Although you want to encourage your child to eat a variety of foods, he is most unlikely to suffer physically because he is going through a faddy phase for a few months. In fact, a fussy eater is likely to be socially handicapped – because mothers of other children may avoid inviting him to share a meal with them – long before he comes to any risk of physical harm.

Keep eating between meals to a minimum. If your child does need something more than a piece of raw vegetable or fruit to keep him going between meals, plan these gap-fillers so that they are like a mini meal. For example, give him a sandwich or a piece of bread and a glass of milk rather than biscuits or a packet of crisps. Then if he is not as hungry at mealtimes, you can still be assured that he has eaten a nutritious mix.

Read and get to understand food labels so that you have a clear idea of what you are feeding your family. Reading a food label is as important in choosing manufactured foods as the look, feel and smell are in judging fresh foods. On the list of ingredients all the contents, except water, have to be declared in descending order of weight. If sugar is the first item listed on a label, for example, it means there is more sugar in the product than any other ingredient. Remember, too, that although a product may state that it contains no artificial preservatives, it may still contain other additives, such as flavourings and colourings. Many products also state their nutritional composition, so you can compare such information as the fat content and calorie value of different brands of low-fat foods.

As you become a better informed consumer you will find it easier to decide which products are made with good quality ingredients and which are not; whether to buy a wholemeal loaf that will last a bit longer because it has a preservative or one that is preservative-free but may go mouldy before it is finished; whether a yoghurt with a low-calorie sweetener is preferable to one sweetened with sugar or to a less sweet one with real fruit.

Healthy choices in the family diet

Food	Healthy choice
Dairy products	
Milk	Skimmed or semi-skimmed milk*.
Hard cheeses	Types labelled low-fat; Edam; or use smaller quantities of a strong-flavoured cheese.
Soft and cream cheeses	Cottage cheese, ricotta, curd cheeses, fromage frais, types labelled low-fat. Camembert type cheeses are medium-fat.
Flavoured and fruit yoghurts	Yoghurts with only fruit added.
Cream	Substitute whole-milk yoghurts, which have less than half the fat of single cream and a quarter to one-third the fat of double cream.
Fats	
Butter and margarine	Low-fat spreads (but take care you don't spread them twice as thick); margarines labelled high in polyunsaturated fatty acids.
Other cooking fats	Soya, sunflower or corn oils; solid cooking fats labelled high in polyunsaturated fatty acids.
Preserves	
Jams	Low-sugar jams or pure fruit spreads
Meats, poultry and fish	
Beef, lamb, pork	Lean cuts. Roast, grill or fry meat in a non-stick pan without extra fat if possible, which allows fat to escape so that it can be drained off. Liver and kidney are generally lean.
In stews and casseroles	Substitute pulses, such as butter beans, baked beans or chick peas, for some of the meat and add plenty of vegetables to increase the fibre content and help reduce fat.

* Children under five with a poor appetite are advised not to have low-fat milk unless by getting fewer calories from it, they are made hungrier for other foods and so make up the shortfall in calories.

Healthy choices in the family diet (cont.)

Food	Healthy choice
Mince	Average mince is 16 per cent fat, so choose lean varieties. Fat can be skimmed off when cold or the mince can be simmered in water for 10 minutes and the liquid drained off before preparing the dish.
Bacon and ham	Cut off fat or pick lean varieties. These are all salty, whether smoked or sweet-cured.
Poultry	Chicken is a lean meat provided the skin is removed before grilling or casseroling and any lumps of fat inside the carcass are removed before roasting. Turkey is even leaner.
Meat products	Canned meats are often very fatty, so instead buy slices of cooked joints of meat from the delicatessen counter, where you can see how much fat there is. The colour of comminuted, processed meats can often disguise their fat content. There are low-fat varieties of sausages and pâtés, but they may still have much the same salt content. Choose vegetable pâtés and nut, bean and seed spreads, such as houmous, tahini and peanut butter. Choose hamburgers, sandwiches made with lean fillings and chicken joints instead of meat pies and sausage rolls.
Fish	Any kind, but preferably not fried or in batter, and not canned in oil unless very well drained.
Vegetables Green and yellow	Fresh or frozen. Canned vegetables lose some of their nutritional value during processing and often have salt and sugar added.
Baked beans	Low-sugar and low-salt varieties are available, but don't spurn the traditional varities, as baked beans are

Food	Healthy choice
	one of the few forms of pulses popular with children.
Potatoes	Serve boiled, mashed or roasted in the minimum of fat without basting. Remember, generous knobs of butter or margarine can be the undoing of an excellent food. Fill baked potatoes with sweetcorn, low-fat cheese, salad, baked beans or chopped raw onion as a change. Thick-cut oven chips are less fatty than thin-cut or deep-fried varieties.
Fruit	Serve fresh fruit, whole or chopped up and mixed with fruit juice, or fruit canned in natural juice, not syrup.
Cereal products Flour	Wholemeal flour or, if you find this too heavy, half white and half wholemeal.
Bread	Wholemeal preferably, though any bread is excellent food.
Rice and pasta	Brown and wholemeal varieties are better, though 'white' varieties are good too.
Sweet pastries and cakes	Buns, scones and teacakes are less fatty (unless thickly spread with butter!) and less sugary than biscuits, iced cakes and pies. Fruit cakes have as much sugar as other cakes but much more fibre.
Savoury pastry dishes	Use a potato topping as in shepherd's pie, or serve stews on a chunk of bread instead of pastry.
Breakfast cereals	Wholegrain, unsweetened varieties or porridge oats. Wean children off pre-sweetened breakfast cereals by giving them the familiar packet but mixing the contents with the unsweetened equivalent; for example, plain cornflakes and sugar-coated cornflakes.
Desserts	Fruit fools made of fruit purée with custard or yoghurt instead of instant pudding mixes; fruit juice set with

Healthy choices in the family diet (cont.)

Food	Healthy choice
	gelatine or jelly crystals without added colouring, instead of commercial jellies; ice lollies made from fruit juice; fruit crumbles with a topping of breadcrumbs, crushed digestive biscuits and/or porridge oats; summer puddings and charlottes made with bread or breadcrumbs instead of flour and fat mixtures.
Sauces and dressings	Low-sugar, low-salt varieties of tomato ketchup or tomato purée thinned with a dash of vinegar and water; low-fat varieties of salad cream; mix mayonnaise half and half with plain low-fat yoghurt for a lighter product with a good flavour; non-oily varieties of French dressing; use lemon or orange juice to add a tang to many salads.
Salt	Instead of relying on salt all the time, use lemon juice, herbs, spices and garnishes of raw, chopped vegetables like onion, peppers and parsley. Have a shaker with a single small hole or a salt grinder so that you end up with less salt 'per sprinkle'.
Snacks	Low-fat, low-salt crisps; bread and bread sticks; crisp rolls; sticks of carrot, courgette and celery; cucumber chunks; cauliflower florets; cubes of cold meat or cheese; frozen banana slices (spread on a tray and take out of the freezer 5 minutes before serving).
	Dried fruit is a good source of fibre, but is also rich in sugar and so can be harmful to teeth if eaten as a snack.
Drinks	Fruit juices, diluted with plain water or sparkling mineral water instead of fizzy drinks or squashes; milk; milk shakes made with orange juice, banana or other fruit purée; water.

Chapter 9

The overweight child and the underweight teenager

A chapter on overweight may seem strange in a book about children who don't eat, but a fat child is no less likely than a slim one to have or have had eating problems such as food fads and poor appetites in his early years. Indeed, if a small appetite has led to a child being encouraged to eat anything he likes – such as a diet of biscuits and sweet drinks – and the child, in fact, thrives on relatively few calories, he may become fat because he is consuming more calories than his body really needs and can burn up.

Parents are not necessarily the first people to notice that their child is overweight. Although you might think his puppy fat is rather charming, you may discover that his classmates consider him fat. The consequences can be mortifying, and the child who is a teased figure of fun may become unhappy and withdrawn or an aggressive little bully in response. An overweight child's problem needs to be tackled, but does not have an easy or speedy solution. Trying to put your child on a slimming diet can be very hard for you as well as for him. Accepting that your child is overweight may lead you to ask yourself to what extent it is your fault, and putting him on a diet may seem like a form of punishment to a child who is already feeling sensitive because of his size. In the case of a girl approaching puberty, you might worry that a child who is encouraged to slim may develop what is popularly, but somewhat inaccurately, called the slimmers' disease – anorexia nervosa.

Causes of overweight

When a person consumes more calories than his body can use, his body stores the excess as fat and he gains weight. Comparing how much your child eats with other children or the amounts suggested on the labels of baby food products does not tell you whether he is eating too much or too little. There can be huge variations in the amounts of food children eat. For example, some two-month-old babies consume as many calories as some two-year-olds, and some children eat twice as much as other children of an identical age and size. It is clear that what and how much a child eats are not the only factors determining his weight.

The amount a child needs to eat – his energy requirement – is determined by his size, his rate of growth and his level of activity. For example, immediately after birth, a baby has a very rapid rate of growth and his level of activity is measured by how wakeful he is. After three months the growth rate begins to slow down and he may become less wakeful, so he needs proportionately fewer calories. When he starts to become mobile in the second half of the first year, the increase in activity causes his appetite to pick up again. Since babies vary enormously in size, degrees of wakefulness, speed of growth and the age at which they start to crawl, their requirements for food, or more specifically calories, vary enormously.

Although this explains why children need to eat different amounts of food to maintain a normal weight, it does not explain why some children eat more than they need and, as a result, are overweight. A popular explanation – or at least one offered by many families with an overweight child – is that overweight 'runs in the family', it is an inherited condition for which little can be done. However, experts on obesity point out that very few of the children who are overweight have a genetic, chronic disorder of the endocrine glands. The majority of children who are overweight are so because they have eaten more calories than their bodies need. The reason that overweight often runs in families is because families tend to share eating habits, good and bad alike. Changing to a healthier diet – one that is low in fat and sugar and high in fibre, fruits and vegetables – to help a child to lose weight could be beneficial to the entire family.

Helping a child lose weight

Changing to a healthy diet

The principal objectives in helping a child to slim are to prevent any further weight gain until his height has 'caught up' in proportion to his weight and to teach him new eating habits. If he tends to eat lots of snacks and small meals, then he – and maybe you as well – need to learn that he should not expect his tummy to feel full all the time and that he will not suffer if there are times during the day when he feels hungry and has to wait for a meal.

If your child eats little between meals and eats regular-sized meals with little variation in appetite, it may be that he never really feels hungry but has learnt to find room for whatever is put in front of him. If he had a poor appetite when he was younger, you may not have stopped the habit of trying to encourage him to eat more or of looking for foods that will entice him to eat. He may be anxious to please and knows that a clean plate gives you satisfaction. In this case help him learn to recognize when he has had enough, and to distinguish between eating because he is hungry and eating for any other reason. You can help him become more independent by encouraging him to serve himself. Reassure him that you will be quite happy if he takes only a small helping, but be careful that you don't ask other members of the family to finish any leftovers, thus encouraging them to develop a weight problem! If you cannot bear waste or find leftovers a nuisance, try deliberately cooking larger quantities with the intention of providing a second meal. Before serving, you can divide the amount prepared in two to avoid the temptation of extra-large first helpings or seconds, then add the leftovers from the serving dishes to the unused portions and freeze them until you want to use them at another meal. In this way you may get used to welcoming leftovers.

In order to lose weight a child does not have to leave a meal feeling hungry, but has to fill up on bulky low-calorie foods such as bread, potatoes, fruit and vegetables rather than on fatty meats and cheese, and sugar-laden desserts and snack foods, which are high in calories, but often are not filling, which is why it is so easy to eat too much of them. There are plenty of healthier, more filling alternatives. For example instead of chips you could serve a large baked potato stuffed with sweet corn or baked beans or dressed with a low-fat mayonnaise. Instead of spaghetti bolognaise (made with fatty mince), you could serve pasta with a cheese sauce made from skimmed milk and low-fat cheddar. Instead of a breakfast of cornflakes and white toast and marmalade, you could serve a wholewheat cereal and wholemeal toast with a low-fat spread and a reduced-sugar jam. High-fibre foods tend to have a high water content, so they are more filling and lower in calories. You can also serve low-calorie squashes and soft drinks, which have been sweetened with an artificial sweetener rather than sugar. How much attention you draw to the way you modify the foods he eats will depend on how much he wants to slim. If he is very concerned about his weight, he may appreciate your constructive help rather than reassurances that he is just cuddly.

If you have difficulty in acknowledging that your child has a weight problem, you may also be deluding yourself about how much he actually eats and drinks during the day. Even if he is not eating large portions at meals, he may be nibbling frequently. It can be instructive to make a note every time he has something to eat or drink, however trivial, over a period of three to four days, including a weekend. You could do the same for yourself and the rest of the family. By becoming more aware of the role food plays in your lives you may be able to pinpoint the times when food is being eaten but isn't really being noticed. For example, have you got into the habit of buying him a packet of crisps on the way home from school; does he nibble bananas or biscuits while he is watching television; are you still offering him whole milk as a drink with his meals? It needs only a regular input of a small number of unnecessary calories each day to make a child put on more weight than he should.

Exercise

Changing or modifying the diet is only one way of helping a child to slim. At the same time you need to ensure that he takes plenty of exercise. Young children should be highly active, skipping, roller skating, riding a bike, running or climbing. Think about how active your child usually is and whether he plays quietly rather than vigorously. Being overweight can slow a child down and always coming last in races or having difficulty jumping over the gym apparatus can be humiliating. A child soon learns to find ways of avoiding such public exposure of his inadequacies. A child doesn't have to be an expert at any sport, but should get pleasure from making his body work hard. If he finds difficulty coping with team sports or competitive games, encourage him to take up activities that aren't competitive and that he enjoys. You may have to get involved too, for example, accompanying him on bike rides, taking him to ice skating classes, swimming or simply throwing a ball with him each day.

Whatever activity your child pursues, help him set realistic, attainable goals. For example, he could aim to skip up to twenty, gradually building to a hundred; he could gradually extend the distance of bicycle rides until he can go, say, a mile; or he can try to increase the number of times he can hit a ball with a bat. Attaining goals, however small, and building on them will be good for his health, his shape and his morale.

Boosting self-confidence

Fat children can feel desperately shy about their size, as can children who are shorter or taller than their friends and classmates. Since there is nothing you can do about your child's height and it will take a bit of time to do something about his weight, help him find something he feels will gain the respect of his classmates. If he tends to get bullied, it may help to send him to judo or karate classes where he can be taught skills that will make him confident that he can defend himself, and that may also impress other children. If he enjoys music, he might like to learn to play an instrument or to dance. He could join a club where he would have the opportunity to learn a hobby thoroughly.

Boys and girls – particularly those who are embarrassed by their size or shape – should be encouraged to have pride in their appearance. Your child may have no inclination to always have a clean face and combed hair but he probably enjoys wearing certain sorts of clothes. Even if he is not fashion conscious, he may appreciate a well-turned-out sports kit. If taking your child clothes shopping is a recipe for disaster, you could at least discuss outfits in catalogues and magazines with him so that you can buy clothes he finds attractive and comfortable.

Perhaps most importantly, you need to give your child time to talk to you each day. A child who feels unhappy or confused needs support. This does not mean trying to protect him from the difficulties of life, but giving him opportunities to be listened to without being interrupted and the security of knowing that what he thinks and feels matters to someone else. If he feels that his opinions and thoughts are carefully considered, it will help give him much-needed confidence to face the many trials and tribulations of growing up.

Anorexia nervosa

Being fat may be distressing, but most parents probably worry more about a child, particularly a daughter, who is excessively thin. Adolescent girls, on the other hand, may regard being too thin as less of an evil than being too fat. Anorexia nervosa is a disorder that results in excessive weight loss. In almost all cases it occurs only after puberty and affects mainly adolescent girls and young women. Although adolescence is outside the age range of this book, anorexia deserves a mention to distinguish it from more common eating problems and to indicate what might be done to prevent it.

A girl suffering from anorexia has a dread of being fat and a fear of putting on weight. To reach what she considers a desirable weight, which she regularly revises downward, she will progressively reduce her consumption of not only what are commonly considered fattening foods, but also all other foods. She may also exercise excessively and take laxatives and diuretics. Some girls develop a related disorder called bulimia nervosa, which is characterized by binge, or uncontrollable, eating from time to time and followed by self-induced vomiting. Anorexia results in a very low body weight, which causes a girl's menstrual periods to cease and can be fatal.

The typical anorexic is a middle-class female aged between 15 and 25. She may possibly, but not necessarily, have been overweight when younger or have had food fads throughout much of her childhood (anorexics often report that as children they were teased about their weight or their appetite); be involved in some sort of physically demanding training, such as ballet or athletics, that requires her to keep a close watch on her weight; or have parents who also have experienced some sort of eating problem or weight disorder, who are artistic or whose work involves them in the preparation of food. Like all anorexics, she feels under considerable pressure, and not just the stress of a tremendously strained relationship with her parents brought about by her condition.

Adolescence can be a time of acute stress. At this age young people have to cope with dramatic physical and emotional changes; the pressures of taking important exams; the prospect of finding a job, starting work and leaving home; and relationships (or lack of them) with the opposite sex. They may feel insecure as they face independence and adult responsibilities. An adolescent girl who lacks confidence and cannot cope with these pressures and responsibilities will clutch at anything that makes her feel she has some control over herself and her life. If she is successful at slimming, and therefore feels it gives her this control, she will be encouraged to continue.

Her peer group may be a source of both pressure and support. Being one of the crowd is particularly important during adolescence and a girl may think that by slimming she will achieve an ideal figure that will make her popular with her peers. Slimming is also an activity that a group of girls can share and an anorexic may report that her friends support her in her efforts to be thin.

The anorexic uses slimming to cope with her stress and her fears of adult life. And if she did not slim, she would simply find another way of 'coping' – for example, by taking drugs, drinking, smoking or becoming pregnant. You can help your child go through adolescence without becoming one of its casualties. As she is growing up, even before she becomes a teenager, don't be over-protective, but encourage her to try new experiences and support her in making her own decisions so that she grows in confidence and resourcefulness.

Chapter 10
The allergic child

Much publicity has been given to the subject of food allergies. Some reports have suggested that as many as 20 per cent of children may suffer from allergies to foods at any one time.[1] Because of such publicity and the fact that allergies to foods are known to be most common in children under seven (after this age substances like pollen, household dust and animal fur are the more usual irritants), it is almost impossible to discuss any symptoms or problems without someone suggesting that an allergy may be the cause. The answer then seems to be relatively simple – find the cause of the allergy, remove it and the problem will go away.

It is at this point that the problems can really begin. Investigating the cause of an allergy can be like looking for a needle in a haystack in the dark. It is all too easy to find nothing or to come across many misleading possibilities. Many symptoms, such as rashes and spots, vomiting and tummy upsets, are very common in childhood and can have many causes other than allergies. Indeed, there may be no identifiable cause: rashes often come and go, children are very easily sick, and children who complain of 'tummy-aches' often have sore throats or want a bit of extra love and attention.

Even when an allergy is identified, treatment is not necessarily obvious or easy. Children who are allergic to food are often allergic to particularly common foods

[1] A. J. Cant, 'Diet and prevention of childhood allergic disease', *Human Nutrition: Applied Nutrition*, vol. 38A, 1984, pp. 455–68.

that can be difficult to exclude from the diet. If they are allergic to more than one food, the treatment – avoiding these foods – may cause more distress than the allergy itself. Having to have a special diet can be a serious social handicap against which children will often rebel. Eliminating a great many foods can also cause health problems unless care is taken to make adequate nutritional substitutes.

What is an allergy?

Allergy is a term often used loosely to describe virtually any repeated adverse reaction to a particular substance. The accurate, scientific definition of an allergy is that the body's immune system has reacted to a harmless substance, which it ought to recognize as safe, as if it were a foreign organism. The reaction may occur within a few minutes of provocation or several hours later and can affect the skin, or the respiratory, digestive or nervous systems. If the skin is affected, the sufferer may get swellings on the face and lips or a bumpy, itchy rash like nettle-rash, as in urticaria, or an irritating rash that weeps to form crusty patches, as in eczema. If the nose or lungs are affected, a person may have a streaming nose, as in hayfever, or wheezy, difficult breathing, as with asthma. If the guts are affected, severe tummy pains or colic, frequent diarrhoea and a general failure to grow and thrive are the likely symptoms. If the nervous system is affected, severe headaches – often affecting just one side of the head – as in migraine, may be the result, or more rarely, particular behaviour problems may arise, as in the case of children with hyperactivity.

Physical symptoms are just one factor in the diagnosis of allergy. Another indicator is a family history of allergies. There is a strong genetic component in allergies and a child whose mother and father have or have had allergies has been calculated to have a 60 per cent chance of developing allergies, though not necessarily the same kind. A child with only one affected parent has a 30 per cent chance, while if neither of his parents has ever suffered from an allergy his chances of developing an allergy are only 5 per cent. It is also suspected that babies who are given solid foods or even fruit drinks before three months of age in the case of low-risk children and before four to six months in the case of high-risk children are also more likely to develop allergies than babies who are weaned later. Babies have immature digestive systems and their guts may not be sufficiently protected against food particles different from milk.[2]

Fortunately, the allergies that affect babies are not usually very severe, and many children grow out of them. Allergies that develop in older children or in children who have a family history of allergy tend to be more severe. Parents are not always the best judges of the severity of an allergy. Not only does a natural concern for their child often alarm parents more than the situation may, in fact, warrant, but most people haven't seen enough other cases to have a reliable scale against which to measure the severity of their child's symptoms. Doctors, who have this experience and know how bad such symptoms can be, can appear to be belittling parents' worries if they don't explain precisely why there is no cause for alarm.

[2] ibid. and *Food Intolerance and Food Aversion*, A Joint Report of the Royal College of Physicians and the British Nutrition Foundation, London, April 1984.

Hyperactivity

Hyperactivity is another term that is frequently used very loosely; instead of being used accurately to describe a serious behavioural disorder, it is often used to label highly energetic, boisterous and mischievous children who are quite normal but can be very exhausting for parents to manage. Hyperactive children are more than simply highly active. They are children who never seem to settle down to toys, games or activities at the same level as other children of their age. They have been described as always restlessly searching for something – without knowing what – that they can take pleasure in.[3] It is unusual for children under the age of three or four years to be diagnosed as hyperactive, as many toddlers are normally very restless and active.

One-third of the parents in one survey described their children as overactive, which shows how normal it is to have a highly active child. The number of children in Britain whose level of activity may be described as abnormal is thought to be less than 1 per cent. In the United States the number of children labelled as hyperactive is much higher – between 5 and 8 per cent. This apparent difference in incidence is due to differences in definitions of the condition.[4]

Research appears to show that hyperactivity is only rarely affected by what children eat. In the cases where food has been shown to aggravate the condition, usually three or four items have been implicated. Apart from the common foods that are often the cause of allergies, two additives – tartrazine (E102, a yellow food colour) and benzoic acid (E210, a preservative that occurs naturally

---

[3] A sensible, sympathetic book for parents is Dr Eric Taylor's *The Hyperactive Child: A Parent's Guide*, Martin Dunitz, London, 1985.
[4] ibid.

in many edible berries as well as being made syntheti-
cally) – were found to be allergenic in a few children.[5]
However, it needs to be emphasized that in these
studies a child who appeared to be allergic to an additive
was usually also sensitive to one or two ordinary foods.
In addition, individual children were allergic to different food items, which makes it difficult to generalize
about which foods a hyperactive child should avoid.

Treating allergies

Unfortunately, there is as yet no cure for food allergies,
although they may go away of their own accord. What
treatment there is can only prevent or control the worst
of the symptoms. If you think your child has an allergy,
have him examined by a doctor. It is important to
determine whether the symptoms are caused by an
allergy or another disorder that needs treatment.

If an allergy is suspected, it is also important to
determine whether something other than food is the
cause, and if food appears to be the culprit, to try other
remedies or methods of coping before experimenting
with changes in your child's diet. For example, eczema
may be caused by a particular washing powder or by
wearing a particular fabric, such as wool, next to the
skin. If it is caused by a food, the irritation may be eased
by avoiding rough fabrics and extremes of temperature,
and by using an oily or emulsifying ointment to keep the
skin soft and supple.

Many doctors are reluctant to suggest eliminating
foods from the diet – particularly in the case of young
children, among whom small appetites and food fads are
so common – partly because finding the culprit, or

[5] A. J. Cant, 'Food allergy in childhood', *Human Nutrition: Applied
Nutrition*, vol. 39A, 1985, pp. 277–293.

culprits, can be very difficult and partly because cutting out foods a child enjoys and expects as a regular part of his diet may add to his distress. If the allergy is caused by a food of minor importance in the diet, such as strawberries or chocolate, it may be easy to avoid. If, however, the allergy is caused by a major food, such as milk or eggs, that provides many nutrients, doctors often prefer to encourage patients to learn to cope with minor symptoms, reserving alterations to the diet as a last resort for children who are severely affected. In the case of mild allergies, which a child will probably grow out of in a few months or years, a doctor might suggest a mild form of treatment as well as some common sense rules of management.

If the allergy is severe or if a particular food seems a likely cause, a doctor may suggest that you try eliminating it from your child's diet for a period of two weeks; one week can be too short a trial period for foods that cause a delayed reaction. If the symptoms do not show signs of clearing up, it is unlikely that that particular food is causing the problem. However, if the symptoms disappear and the culprit food is an important item in your child's diet, you may be referred to a dietician (in a hospital or attached to an allergy clinic), who will help you work out a suitable alternative diet and advise you on all the food products that may contain the offending item. It can be difficult to avoid seemingly simple foods unless you read food labels very carefully and know what all the terms indicate. For example, milk or eggs are present if any of the following ingredients are listed on the food label: milk, butter, cream, cheese, cheese powder, skimmed milk powder, non-fat milk solids, casein, caseinate, whey, lactalbumin and egg lecithin.

Since children can become tolerant of foods that once provoked a reaction, the dietician will advise you on when to reintroduce the food to see if the allergy has disappeared. This is called a dietary challenge and very often occurs unintentionally, for, unless you are vigilant about reading food labels and never let your child out of your sight, then sooner or later he will help himself or be given the offending food.

Preventing allergies

There is fairly good evidence that allergies can be prevented or, at least, their severity reduced if special care is taken over what babies eat in infancy. This is particularly important in the case of children with a family history of allergies. It is widely believed in medical circles that breast-feeding exclusively (which means no supplements of formula milks or other foods) in the early weeks helps protect against allergies. If breast-feeding is not possible, one of the modified formula milks is a good second best. The proteins – the allergenic constituents – in cow's milk are so altered during the processing that these formulas are believed to be much less likely to set off allergic reactions than unprocessed cow's milk.

Other milks – soya formulas and goat's milk – have also been advocated as safe alternatives to formula milks based on cow's milk. However, soya formula is no less likely than cow's-milk formula to cause an allergy if it is given to a child in the first few weeks of life. In other words, any foreign protein is likely to trigger an allergic response if it is given at a time when the baby's digestive and immune systems are vulnerable. On the other hand, soya formula is a useful alternative for an older baby with a known allergy to cow's milk.

Goat's milk is neither nutritionally adequate for babies under six months nor any less allergenic than cow's milk, and it cannot be guaranteed bacteriologically safe, as it is not subject to the same government regulations as cow's milk.

There have been claims that foods can trigger allergies by being passed to the foetus through the placenta or to the baby through breast milk. There is little evidence that eating or avoiding specific foods during pregnancy affects the development of allergies in a baby. If you are breast-feeding and your baby develops symptoms of an allergy, it may be worth excluding eggs and milk – the foods that are most likely to cause most allergies – from your diet for two weeks. If your baby's symptoms do not improve, there is no point in your continuing; in trials only one-quarter of infants with eczema and one-third of thse with colic showed any signs of improvement.[5]

If your baby does get better during this period, you will need professional dietetic advice on what to eat instead of the offending foods. If you have been eliminating dairy products, you will need an alternative source of calcium, as in the early months of his life your baby takes considerable amounts of calcium from you through breast-feeding. To maintain your milk supply you will also almost certainly need to make up the calories lost by excluding these foods, as there is little to be gained from swapping the cries of an itchy or colicky baby for those of a hungry one.

If your baby runs a high risk of developing allergies, feed him only breast milk for at least four, and preferably six, months. In order to satisfy his appetite you will need to feed him more frequently and for longer than if he were being weaned. When you start feeding him solids, introduce them one at a time, giving each one daily for a week before starting another. Some foods are

[5] Ibid.

more likely to cause allergies than others, so introduce the least allergenic types first, as shown in the chart below.

If after the introduction of a new food, your baby develops a red, itchy rash or has loose, unusually smelly, watery stools, stop giving him that food. And while you are taking such care of his diet, remember to avoid other known irritants, such as wool next to the skin, house dust, talcum powder, animal fur, scented soaps and lotions, and biological washing powders.

Order of foods for weaning

First foods
Milk-free baby rice mixed with water or breast milk
Puréed root vegetables, such as potatoes, carrots, swede and parsnip
Puréed apple, pear and banana
Other puréed vegetables, including peas, lentils, beans and leeks
Other cereals, such as oats and maize, but not wheat
Lamb, turkey and then other meats

From 8 months
Wheat-based cereals

From 9 months
Citrus fruits and citrus fruit drinks

From 10 months
Fish and yoghurt; boiled cow's milk can be given, but milk feeds should be breast milk or soya formula. If boiled cow's milk is tolerated, butter, cheese and infant food formulas containing dried milk can be included in the diet.

From 12 months
Eggs

Chapter 11
A last word

This book has tried to cover the full range of eating problems. After reading it I hope you have discovered that eating problems are not only common, but that they are also not so surprising in the context of your child's development as a whole. By understanding the stages of your child's development you can try to nip eating problems in the bud or help him to grow out of the awkward stages, so that he learns to enjoy good, healthy food.

I have suggested a number of ways for coping with each of the eating problems you may encounter so you can choose the ones that fit in with your general approach to your child's upbringing. You have to carefully work out exactly what changes you want to make and be prepared to stick firmly to your decision. Your chances of success are probably better if you make changes gradually, so that both you and your child can get used to them at a comfortable pace. A sudden turning over of a new leaf can be not only exciting, but also alarming. It may be much harder to enforce and provoke a child's resistance.

If a particular approach does not show any signs of success after a week or so, try something different, but take the initiative rather than permitting your child effectively to dictate what is to happen. For example, if you decide that he will get no pudding until he has eaten at least half his first course but he still will not eat more than a couple of spoonfuls, don't give in after the third or fourth day; your child's persistence is likely to be more enduring than your patience. Instead, if you cannot bear him going without anything at a meal, wait until the next meal and tell him you will give him his pudding – some fruit, not a sweet – to eat as a starter or as a 'vegetable' if he prefers. You can then tell him he has had his pudding, but at the same time show him that he has actually obeyed the rules you have made – albeit in the form of a compromise.

Sometimes a problem will get worse before it gets better. When a child finds he is not getting his own way it is hardly surprising if he objects. By being firm and calm, and not engaging in a battle, you will eventually make him realize that making a fuss will not get him what he wants. If you are not sure you will be able to stick to your guns, set yourself a small target before you tackle the bigger issues.

Useful addresses

When requesting information from the following organizations, send a large, stamped, self-addressed envelope.

Anorexic Aid
    The Priory Centre
    11 Priory Road
    High Wycombe
    Buckinghamshire, HP13 6SL
    Tel: 0494 21431
Aims to give support and information to sufferers of anorexia and bulimia nervosa and their families through correspondence or meetings of self-help groups.

Child Growth Foundation
    2 Mayfield Avenue
    London W4 1PW
    Tel: 01 995 0257 or 01 994 7625
Offers parental support and information as well as raising money to support specialists and institutions caring for children with growth disorders.

Hyperactive Children's Support Group
    The Secretary
    71 Whyke Lane
    Chichester
    West Sussex PO19 2LD
Helps parents cope with hyperactive children and supports research into, and gives publicity to, hyperactivity in children.

National Childbirth Trust
  9 Queensborough Terrace,
  London W2 3TB
  Tel: 01 221 3833
Offers antenatal classes, support with breast-feeding, encouragement with parenthood after the baby is born. Local branches and groups, and a network of breast-feeding counsellors throughout the UK.

National Eczema Society
  Tavistock House north,
  Tavistock Square,
  London WC1H 9SR
  Tel: 01 388 4097
Encourages research into, and spread of information about, eczema. Local groups for people with eczema and their relatives.

Index